HE GAVE ME
COMFORT

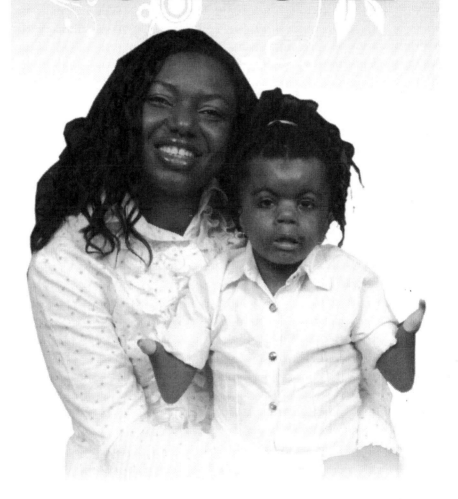

Eyum Ocheola-Oki

Copyright © 2011, 2012 by Eyum Ocheola-Oki

Published by:

Impact Life Publisher

62A Airlie Heights,

Lucan, CO.Dublin

Republic of Ireland

Email: info@hegavemecomfort.com

ISBN: 978-0-9574241-0-4

Cover Design by:
FirmWord, Ireland.
Tel: +353871311772

Table of Contents

DEDICATION

To the Almighty God who never makes mistakes in His work of creation.

To the Lord Jesus Christ who is my advocate for grace

To the Holy Spirit who is my comforter

To every Parent and Carer of children with special needs who has not given up on them.

SPECIAL THANKS

First and foremost to the husband of my youth, Pastor Enoch Enenche Ocheola-Oki. Your love and support has been overwhelming. Apart from being a husband, you are also my friend, coach, motivator and strong pillar. This book is as a result of your constant pruning of my life over the last 17 years.

To my kids, Ochanya, Olijeh & Eyum(Jnr). You gals are always there for me, loving and helping me in whatever way you can. And to Grace, you are so good and understanding, happily accepting whatever we have to offer you.

To my spiritual father, Reverend Simeon Afolabi. There are many instructors, but very few fathers. I cannot forget how you stuck close during those devastating moments, even though I was in a faraway land, you regularly checked on me by your constant phone calls. For your unquantifiable input to this book, I say thank you so much.

To Pastor Tunde Adebayo-Oke and Dr Elizabeth Omole for taking time out of your very busy schedules to read the manuscript and make your invaluable inputs. May the Lord abundantly reward you for the good seed sown into my life.

To Sister Yinka Sanni. You are truly a child of God and a faithful servant of our Lord, Jesus Christ. In a foreign land where I knew nobody, you positioned yourself as a sister that stood by me and helped me to regain my strength.

To the government of Ireland, the host of medical personnel and everyone that has worked with Grace at one point or the other. You guys have shown me that Grace is not just my baby, but 'our' baby because of your overwhelming support. Fiona Lyons, you went beyond your normal call of duty as a medical social worker at the time of Grace's birth. May my God abundantly reward you.

To my parents, Hon. Eigege Ejiga & Mrs Grace Ejiga; the upbringing you gave to me helped me to endure tough times. And Papa, thank you for the gift of writing that you passed to me.

To my entire church family, Kingdom Gospel Centre, Dublin, you guys are too much! You are always there giving your support in season and out of season. Obehi Ebhiemhen, Ochanya Ocheola-Oki and Michelle Keogh for taking your time to do the initial proof-reading of the manuscript; I say thanks a million.

To Lena Maria and Nick Vujicic, for allowing me to use your inspiring stories and photographs in this book. And to all my numerous pastors, friends and family members whose names I cannot all mention here. I appreciate the support every one of you has given to me at one point or the other. God, who is a rewarder, will not forget all your labour of love.

PREFACE

We live in an age of swift news (report) transmission by virtue of technology. But the amazing thing is that most of the reports we get to hear are intimidating, depressing, devastating and heart breaking reports. The world is prone to reporting evil report than good report! I have heard it say that Bad news is good business. When we turn to the television, all we hear and see is intimidating! We turn to the radio and Internet, the same devastating and depressing news still flaunt themselves. Even when we go to our doctors, the reports are still not any better. We still get heart-breaking reports. This is THE WORLD REPORT!

In the midst of all these evil, intimidating reports, what do you do? You can turn to the GOOD NEWS, which is the Bible. There you will find hope in a hopeless situation, uplifting in a depressed situation, direction in a confused situation, and light when all seems dark! This is known as the WORD REPORT!

As free moral beings living in this world, we are therefore faced daily with two options of report from which to believe - THE WORLD REPORT and THE WORD REPORT. You have the onus to choose which option to believe. Would you believe the World report that can destroy you, or would you rather believe the Word report that is good and would build you up, and give you a hope and a future.

This book aims to encourage you to tune yourself to the Word Report. In it, you will receive comfort and solutions to your problems. Even when the report of the world has concluded that there is no hope, things will always change for good when you encounter the Word report.

FOREWORD

By the time I was asked to do the foreword to this book I had about three or four other manuscripts lying on my desk waiting for similar attention. This became a challenge to me, because I could not figure out where in the world I would get time to do this. I could have asked someone to do the reading, give me the summary and then scribble something down. But I have a rule: I usually don't like to do foreword for a work I have not read (possibly twice). Two things became the inspiration for me to accept the task. First is my personal knowledge of the enormous problem the Ocheola-Okis faced when Grace was born. I was one of the first few individuals they contacted to break what you would call a bad news. Because of distance all I could do then was to offer prayers. But when I visited them in Dublin in 2009 and 2010 I had first-hand opportunity to see Grace. The other thing that spurred me was the richness of the material itself. After what seemed to be a millennium I finally moved to at least gloss over some aspects of the work with the aim of facing it later. From that first moment I could not put it down. I could see life-changing lessons poured into the pages of this book in pure emotion and utmost candour.

Things sometime happen in life that defies all explanation. All the more confounding is it when bad things (by human standards) happen to good people. We become confused because we cannot reconcile our circumstance to the fact that God is love and is busy promoting the best for us in life. In such situations all we are left with is our attitude, how we choose to respond. It has become popular to hear that life is not so much of what happens, but how we handle what comes our path. The Ocheola-Okis did not choose what happened when Grace was born; but I am happy they have taken everything in their stride and are making the most of their life's circumstance.

As I pored through this material several things impressed me greatly. I have come to appreciate the fact that a united, loving family front can scale through the toughest of hurdles. Everyone in the family rally round to support another. I believe the emotional bond exhibited, by which unblemished love is given to this special member of the family, will play a definite role in whatever final miracle God is bringing to Grace. On another note I see how our greatest problems have underneath them great prospects. By the way, except Grace came the way she did you will definitely not have this book in your hand; at least not in this format. She has not only made this book possible but has also opened other avenues of serving God and His people. When a problem has become a source of solving other problems then you can be sure God has started to work everything out for good. I see this happening already.

What you have in your hand is not some theories propounded in some social science laboratory. It is step-by-step account of how a mother has continued to cope with what would be daunting to others. She has not only revealed her secrets in dealing with the tough issues of life but also presented several other cases in and out of the Bible. This book will not only strengthen you to deal with any immediate challenge you may have right now, but it will also equip you for the future. I am sure that by the time you are through reading the material you will be in a position to surmount any challenge, no matter how formidable.

Simeon O. Afolabi
Firstlove Assembly,
Portharcourt, Nigeria.

INTRODUCTION

GOD IS A COMFORTER

"Blessed be the God and Father of our Lord Jesus Christ, the father of mercies and God of all comfort, who comforts us in all our tribulation, that we may be able to comfort those who are in any trouble, with the comfort with which we ourselves are comforted by God."
II Corinthians 1: 3-4

Indeed, God is a comforter!
I write this book based on the comfort that I have received from God and the hope He has given me in a seemingly hopeless situation. I came to Ireland in January, 2004 pregnant with our fourth child. Shortly after I arrived, things started happening at a faster rate than I could cope with or understand. On the evening of 26th January, 2004; I was rushed to the Rotunda Hospital after my water had broken. On examination by doctors in

the emergency unit, I was given several reasons why an emergency caesarean section had to be carried out on me.

The first shock I had when I saw my baby was that she was very tiny, weighed about 2.08kg and looked somehow funny. The first striking contrast between Grace and any other baby was that her upper arm was very short, bent upwards from the elbow and very tight; and she had just one finger on each arm. She was so weak and feeble, the doctors said had there been a little delay before the section, she would not have made it. Even after her delivery, she was still very weak and could not tolerate food. Almost everyone thought Grace was going to die.

After series of tests and examinations on her, she was diagnosed with a condition known as Cornelia de Lang syndrome (for details about this condition, you can visit: www.corneliadelang.org); a very rare medical condition whose prognosis is not known (they claim it just happens), neither does medical science have a cure for it. It is attributed to some genetic disorders.

To say I was devastated is an understatement. Sleep eluded me for days. Where did things go wrong? What does the future hold for me and this child? What......? How.........? Why...........? So many questions, so many puzzles, no satisfactory answer! It was like my world had come to a standstill. In the midst of my tears, confusion and hopelessness, I turned to the Lord, the God of all comfort; and He alone was able to comfort me. When I did not know what to do, at least I knew where to go! KNOW WHERE TO GO, WHEN YOU DON'T KNOW WHAT TO DO!

When I turned to the Lord for comfort, He gave me the following words:

- The Lord told me that this situation has happened that His name would be glorified (John 9:3).
- The Lord told me that he allowed this to happen "that He might humble me and test me, to do me good in the end" Deuteronomy 8:16b.

To tell you the truth, I am already seeing the goodness of the Lord in this situation. A lot of blessings have come my way and indeed the entire family! She has brought uplifting to us!! Although all that I believe God for, in her life are not yet manifested physically, but I can tell you that she is doing tremendously well. Her GP (General Practitioner), the Professor of Genetics, and all the host of consultants that saw her when she was born; and have seen her in recent times, have all exclaimed one statement: "This girl has proved us wrong, we thought she would not survive, but she is doing better than we expected."

Do you know that since Grace was born, **no single surgery** (whether major or minor) has been performed on her? Most children with this condition live in and out of hospitals, yet my child has never spent up to one full week in the hospital since her discharge after she was born. Most children with this condition cannot eat orally (that is through the mouth), they have to be fed through tubes, yet my own child gobbles everything through her mouth. Most children with the condition are on at least one constant medication, but Grace is not. I could go on and on.

Do you know what has kept this girl thriving? Her dad and I (as her parents) have chosen to believe the report of the Lord. When I gave birth to this child, I went to the bible again to see what God says about children and this is what I found:

- Children are a **gift** from the Lord, they are a reward from Him. Psalms 127:3 (NLT)
- The blessing (**gift**) of the Lord makes one rich, And He adds no sorrow with it. Proverbs 10:22
- I and the children that the Lord has given to me are for signs and wonders. Isaiah 8:18.

Believing these scriptures (and many more) has given me hope; wiped away my tears and indeed, I have been comforted!!! The amazing and interesting thing is that the more I choose to trust God, the more of His goodness I see.

What challenges are you confronted with right now? Is it an ill-health? Is it some form of lack in the area of finance, material possessions or the fruit of the womb? Or is it even a very rare situation that I may not even be aware of? Then know that, that is the more reason why you need to believe God's report! You are not alone in what you are passing through. If you will choose to believe the report of the Lord, He will use that same challenge to glorify His name and lift you up.

CHAPTER 1

WHERE COULD THINGS HAVE GONE WRONG?

There was a puzzled look on their faces, and quickly she was taken to another room.

This was on one fateful Monday evening, around 8.18pm on the 26th of January, 2004 to be precise. I had been rushed by an ambulance to the emergency section of The Rotunda Hospital in Dublin at about 6p.m. My water had broken prior to this time and I was in serious pains. I had to wait for a while because there were so many people waiting to be seen at the emergency section. As the pain was getting unbearable, I approached a nurse and asked whether I can have a pain reliever. She simply told me that I cannot take any medication until I had been examined by the doctor. And then finally I was called in by the doctor.

On examining me, he requested some other medical personnel to join him in the examination. I was then told that they had to carry out an emergency caesarean section on me due to these reasons:

- The baby was lying transverse (Bridge or across)
- There was a reduced variability of the CTG
- I was only 2cm dilated
- And the baby was already very distressed and if nothing is done immediately, she may not make it.

I was then carried to the theatre for the surgery. They asked me if I wanted to be given a general anaesthetic that would knock me off completely or if I wanted to see the operation being performed, in that case, I would be given an epidural anaesthetic where I would be awake and yet feel no pain and see the surgery being performed. The latter option intrigued me as I have never had any surgery whatsoever carried out on me. I thought it would be cool (interesting) to watch as your tummy is being opened to bring out the baby. I have had three children before now, and all the deliveries were normal.

The surgery went on smoothly and I saw when the baby was brought out of me. My first shock was that the baby looked so tiny and somehow funny. She was immediately taken to another room, and after that followed a series of questions from the medical team. The questions were so numerous that I could hardly remember them all, but they were questions like - Do you have **this** condition, and **that** condition and this **other** condition in your family? They were actually mentioning the names of the conditions most of which I have never heard of. All my answers were NO. One question I will never forget was that asked by the midwife: Do you want to see the baby?

It was at this point that I got really scared. Why would she ask me if I wanted to see my own baby? What kind of baby did I have that would warrant her asking me this question? The midwife then went on to explain to me that there were some complications with the baby and that she has some missing limbs. Her description of the baby was very scary. I was so frightened that I could not answer in the affirmative; I did not have the courage to see and embrace my baby that night. I was then taken to the ward and the baby was taken to the Intensive Care Unit (ICU). Despite the surgery and the anaesthetics that were given to me, I could hardly sleep that night. I lay there in pains throughout the night weeping and wondering - What have I given birth to? Where could things have gone wrong?

The night seemed so long and eventually, the day broke. I actually thought that all the incidents of the previous day were a dream and I wished it was actually a dream! It was when a nurse came to attend to me that I realised that I was not dreaming. I told her I would like to see my baby that morning. A wheel chair was brought for me, and I was wheeled to the intensive care unit where she was. The intensive care unit is on a different floor from the ward. The hospital is a multi-storey building with so many arms. It is said to be over a hundred years old, but it looked very new and immaculate due to renovations and very good maintenance. The usual stink that I know to be associated with hospitals was not there, and I wondered what made the difference between this hospital and most of the hospitals that we have in Africa.

There she was, kept in a glass-like unit with some gadgets all around her. I looked at her and she looked beautiful! She did not look as bad as the midwife had described her to me the previous day. I felt bad that I did not see her the previous day. I held her in my arms and wept uncontrollably, still wondering where things could have gone wrong. After I had quietened down, though my eyes were still wet, I decided to pray and committed her to God's hands. Even though all that was happening was too much for me to take in or even understand, I still thanked God for her because I believe that she is still a gift from Him; remembering the word of God in Psalms 127 verse 3 that says Children are a **gift** from the Lord, and the fruit of the womb is **His reward**. But what I could not understand is why

God would choose to reward us this way, because this did not look like a pleasant reward considering how we as a family have faithfully served Him.

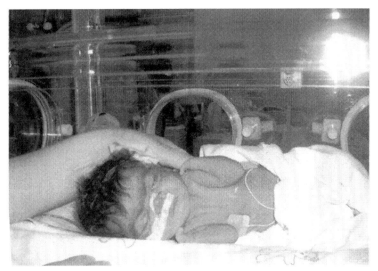

Picture of Grace a few days after she was born

She is our daughter

Shortly after I returned to the ward that morning, my husband rang from Nigeria to find out how I was doing. He was surprised to hear that I had already had the baby. This is because my EDD (Expected Date of Delivery) was towards the end of February, and given that my babies always tend to arrive later than the EDD (at least from my experience in the previous pregnancies), it was quite a shock to him. But he was yet to receive the greatest shock! I was weeping when I answered his call that morning and I just blurted out: Honey, I'm in the hospital, I had the baby last night. That's surprising, he said.   Honey, 'what I gave birth to does not look like a child at all', I said, and I went on to describe the baby. He allowed me to talk, and when I finished, he simply and emphatically said: "She is our daughter".

Although I was not exactly sure what his reaction would be, I must say that I was a bit taken aback by his quick and complete acceptance of the baby. After having our first three daughters, we decided to put a hold on having more children. This pregnancy was not even a planned one. But when we discovered that I was pregnant again, we prayed and hoped that it would be a boy this time; but we not only got a girl, but a severely disabled one. That is why those words "she is our daughter" meant so much to me. Those words went a long way to comfort me and to also help me to accept the baby. She is indeed our daughter! We gave her three names: **Grace** (Believing that the Grace of God will be sufficient to see her through life), **Miracle** (Believing God to manifest his wonder-working power through her life) and **Ehigocho** (this is in our local dialect, meaning 'The Gift of God').

Before I came to Ireland, I did a few scans, but somehow they did not detect any abnormalities with the pregnancy, and if they did, they did not tell me. But somehow I felt that all was not well with the pregnancy. Several times, I have asked my husband to pray for me while I was pregnant and he would lay his hands on my tummy and pray for me and the baby. I believe God was just using this intuition to prepare me for what was ahead.

I resolved not to treat her differently

I determined from the onset that I wasn't going to treat her differently from the way I treated the other children. I was going to love her and raise her in the same way I did the others. I always breast-feed my children exclusively for the first few months until the breast milk alone was no longer sufficient to sustain them; and that was also what I wanted to do for her. But because she was in the ICU, I was told that if I wanted to breastfeed her, I had to express the milk before it could be given to her. This I did, but unfortunately, her system could not tolerate the milk and she had to be placed on a drip. But after a few days, she started to take a little of the breast milk along with the drip, until her intake of milk was high enough and the drip was removed after about a week.

After we were discharged from the hospital, I still tried to continue breastfeeding her, but I discovered that even though she latched onto the breast and gave indications of sucking, my breast milk had begun to dry up and that she did not have a bowel motion in two days. It was at this point that I decided to try her with bottled milk which actually confirmed that although she gave indications of sucking the milk, after 30 minutes of sucking, the milk would still be at the same level. It was real hard work trying to get just a little food into her. Her weight which was 2.08kg when she was born had now dropped to 1.96kg. I had to start praying for her to take in food, and gradually she started taking small amounts such as 10mls at a time, gradually increasing to 30mls, and after about a month, her weight started to pick up gradually.

The Diagnosis

Various Doctors and consultants were called in to examine Grace and they all had an opinion of what they thought her condition was, based on her physical deformity and other features. But a confirmation was needed from an expert in the field of genetics (since they attributed her condition to some genetic disorders). Professor Green, a professor of Genetics was invited from another hospital to come and examine her. After Professor Green's examination, he diagnosed a condition known as Cornelia de Lang syndrome. This condition is said to be very rare, the probability of it occurring in one out of every 40,000 to 100,000 births. The prognosis of this condition they say is not known - they claim that it just happens.

At the time that Professor Green was examining Grace, it happened that I had just stumbled out of the hospital just before his arrival. I had been discharged on that day, although Grace was still in the hospital. Having been told that he will be coming that day, I had waited for a long while for him and when he seem to be running very late, I had to go and sort out my accommodation issue. It was during my short absence that he came and examined Grace. It was on my return to the hospital that I was embraced with the very devastating news of the diagnosis and what it entails. By the time they explained to me some of the woes associated with the condition, I couldn't help but break down again, and I was re-admitted back to the hospital that night. I was made to understand that the physical deformity is only a little fraction of all that the condition entails.

Another appointment was made for us to see Professor Green several weeks later, after which he sent me this letter (see appendix 1 for letter).

CHAPTER 2

PRECEDENCE

"No temptation has overtaken you except such as is common to man; but God is faithful, who will not allow you to be tempted beyond what you are able, but with the temptation will also make the way of escape, that you may be able to bear it."
I Corinthians 10:13

"The temptations in your life are no different from what others experience. And God is faithful. He will not allow the temptation to be more than you can stand. When you are tempted, He will show you a way out so that you can endure. "
I Corinthians 10:13(NLT)

Could a new Specie of humans have started with me? I have never seen or heard of anyone born with missing limbs! This was one of my fears when I gave birth to Grace, but as I was being exposed to information and knowledge, I was liberated from this fear.

There is a law called the 'Law of Precedence'. Lawyers will be very familiar with this law. In the application of this law, a lawyer would seek to establish whether there is a previously handled case similar to the current one he has at hand. If he finds one, he examines the elements of the case, how it was handled and the outcome of it. From there he draws inferences as he handles his current case. Lawyers that apply the law of Precedence cannot but win their cases because they would have convinced the judge beyond all reasonable doubt to make judgment in their favour. I believe the word in 1 Corinthians 10:13 above, is talking about this law of precedence which says that whatever you are faced with right now is not peculiar to you; someone in this life has gone through it before, someone is going through that same situation right now, and someone will still face the same situation in future. So instead of wallowing in self-pity and all the other negative attitudes, you need to start digging into the law of precedence in your particular case. Just know that whatever you are confronted with today is not new, neither is it strange! Men may have given a very high-sounding, jaw-breaking word to qualify or name your situation, but it is not strange. You may never have heard of your kind of situation before, neither have you seen it, but I tell you it is not new.

During my second level education, I had this teacher that always told us the story of a frog in a well. He told us that the frog in a well knows only about its immediate environment (which is the well), and therefore thinks that the whole world is contained in the well. This frog is not aware that there is much life and activities outside that well. Its' confinement has greatly limited its' knowledge and access to information.

Do you know that challenges sometimes confine us like this frog? We often become short-sighted when confronted with challenges. We hardly see beyond it, and think that the whole world ends around our challenges or trying moments. I urge you therefore to begin to apply this law of precedence as you now choose to go for more knowledge and enlightenment about your situation, but please go for positive enlightenment!

Negative Precedence
I realise that there is a culture of precedence that is practiced in medicine in the Western world (developed countries). When a medical condition is diagnosed in a patient, one of the things the medical team does, is to find or search out for someone that earlier had that condition. When they come across someone, they try to link up the two people involved, if they are interested. The only drawback I may say is that their precedence tends

to be towards the negative. They believe they should prepare your mind for the worst case scenario, so that you can know what ailments or problems to expect, and how you may be able to manage them. They believe that having made known to you what to expect, you will be able to condition your mind to accept the situation and live with it. Unfortunately, this is a negative precedence that destroys faith and gives no room for the miraculous and supernatural.

I remember when I gave birth to Grace; the medical team did their findings and discovered that there were a few families in Dublin (Republic of Ireland) that had children with this condition. They asked me if I wanted to meet any of them, but because there were so many negative reports that I had already been told about the condition, I declined. I didn't have the courage to see the negative things I had heard being materialised in someone. It was not until over a year after my daughter was born that I summoned courage to meet with someone that had the condition. This meeting was around mid-2006; and the person I was to meet with was about 18 years of age, although he looked quite small (maybe like a 10-11 year old). The boy didn't have any missing fingers like my daughter, he had all his fingers and other parts of the body complete; but there was a striking resemblance between the two of them. This boy didn't have any words or speech at this age and he was not able to use the sign language either. He was sniffing people like animals would do. I left this meeting with tears in my eyes. Throughout that day, I couldn't help the tears from coming; even when driving and carrying out my chores, the tears continued to pour.

The thought on my mind was: why would God give me a child like this, a child whose behavioural pattern would be very similar to that of an animal? I was brooding over this for the whole day and into the night that I could hardly sleep, until I heard a very sharp rebuke from the Lord asking me: whose report would you believe? I was startled, and I re-echoed the question back to myself. I had reduced myself into believing the world's report; and thinking that my daughter would exhibit the same characteristics I had seen in an older child with the condition; forgetting who I am in Christ. This question revitalised my faith in God and I made up my mind to believe the report of the Lord. The report that says children are a gift from Him; the report that says His gift makes rich and does not add sorrow to it; the report that says I and my children are for signs and wonders; the report that says God will perfect all that concerns me; and so on and so forth. And I heard the Spirit of the Lord speak to my spirit that I would not only believe for myself, but I would also write a book to encourage other people to believe the Lord's report as well. This is why I am writing this book. Negative precedence can be very devastating, so I encourage you not to dwell on them.

Positive Precedence

Your first point of reference when looking for positive precedence should be the Word of God which is the Bible. This is because it is God's manual for living for humans. Anyone that manufactures a product also makes a manufacturer's manual to aid in the use of the product. In the same way, God who has created or manufactured man has also given the Bible as a manual to aid us in living. Therefore when you are confronted with a challenge, the first thing you need do is to look for precedence from the Bible. Ask yourself questions like; has this happened before in the Bible; how did the person(s) involved go through it; and what was their final outcome? This is because all that is written in the Bible is written for us to learn from - "For whatever things were written before were written for our learning, that we through the patience and comfort of the scriptures might have hope." Romans 15:4.

HAS THIS HAPPENED BEFORE?

> *Is there anything of which it may be said,*
> *"See, this is new"? It has already been in*
> *ancient times before us.*
> Ecclesiastes 1:10

History merely repeats itself. It has all been done before. Nothing under the sun is truly new. Sometimes people say, "Here is something new!" But actually it is old; nothing is ever truly new.
Ecclesiastes 1:9-10 (NLT)

There is no challenge you are confronted with right now that is new. It definitely has happened before in ancient times (History), and there also would be a similar case in the Bible.

Like I mentioned earlier on, when I had Grace, one of the reasons why I was so devastated was because I thought a new Specie of humans had begun with me. I had never seen this kind of case before; neither have I read or heard about it before. And as a matter of fact, most of the doctors around me were also seeing the condition for the very first time. It was all so strange! But with information gathered, I later realised that there is a probability of this condition in one of every 40,000 to 100,000 live births. Therefore as strange as this condition was to me and the people around me, it is not new. It has happened in history before.

When I also looked into the Bible, I also found that it has happened even in Bible times before! Of course the name 'Cornelia de Lang Syndrome' is not in the Bible. This is because the condition was named after one female medical doctor (Dr Cornelia de Lang) who did a lot of research on the condition, and because she didn't live in biblical times, her name couldn't have appeared in the Bible. For instance, in the Bible, there is a case of a man with withered hand (Mark 3:1-5), there is a case of someone with impediment of speech (Mark 7:32), and above all, there are series of cases of people born with different kinds of severe disability. For instance, in John 9:1, there is the case of a man that was born blind; In Acts 3:2, there is the case of a man lame from the womb; and in Acts 14:8, there is the case of a man crippled from birth. This settles my own precedence from the Bible. You will agree with me that in all these cases they were all perfected (healed).

A man with withered hand

> While in Capernaum Jesus went over to the synagogue again, and noticed a man there with a deformed hand. Since it was Sabbath, Jesus' enemies watched him closely. Would he heal the man's hand? If he did, they planned to arrest him! Jesus asked the man to come and stand in front of the congregation. Then turning to his enemies he asked, "Is it all right to do kind deeds on Sabbath days? Or is this a day for doing harm? Is it a day to save lives or to destroy them?" But they wouldn't answer him. Looking around at them angrily, for he was

deeply disturbed by their indifference to human need, he said to the man, "Reach out your hand." he did, and instantly his hand was healed!
Mark 3:1-5 (TLB)

The Bible did not tell us here whether the man was born with the deformed hand, or whether it got deformed as a result of an accident or disease. Although a Bible scholar (Marvin Vincent) in Word Studies tells us that the hand probably got deformed as a result of an accident or disease. Anyway, whatever caused the deformity is not as important as the fact that the hand was restored. It was healed and made whole! This is my precedence, that if Jesus restored a withered hand, He can also restore that of my daughter and yours too, as we choose to believe Him. This is because 'Jesus Christ is the same yesterday, today and forever' (Hebrews 13:8).

Deaf and Dumb (speech Impediment) healed
Then they brought to Him one who was deaf and had an impediment in his speech, and they begged Him to put His hand on him. And he took him aside from the multitude, and put His fingers in his ears, and He spat and touched his tongue. Then looking up to heaven, He sighed, and said to him, "Ephphatha," that is, "Be opened." Immediately his ears were

opened, and the impediment of his tongue was loosed, and he spoke plainly. Then He commanded them that they should tell no one; but the more He commanded them, the more widely they proclaimed it. And they were astonished beyond measure, saying, "He has done all things well. He makes both the deaf to hear and the mute to speak."
Mark 7:32-37.

Your case will be the next astonishment to people around you in Jesus name, Amen! Even if the medical report says you cannot speak as a result of your condition, the power that loosed this man's tongue to speak clearly will also loose yours to speak in the mighty name of Jesus, Amen.

The ways of God can sometimes be weird. Can you imagine Jesus spitting, and touching the man's tongue with his saliva? This does not sound very hygienic, but the man got his miracle! I would rather do weird things at the instruction of God to get my miracle than try to be cool and continue in my suffering! Remember the words of the Mary, the mother of Jesus - "Whatever He says to you, do it" (John 2:5). This is the secret to receiving from God. As you believe His word, let your spirit be sensitive to receive instructions from Him; and whatever He tells you to do, just do it even if it doesn't look sensible or rational to do it.

A man blind from birth

Now as Jesus passed by, he saw a man who was blind from birth. And His disciples asked Him, saying, "Rabbi, who sinned, this man or his parents, that he was born blind?" Jesus answered, "Neither this man nor his parents sinned, but that the works of God should be revealed in him.
John 9:1-3

In this case, the man was not just blind, but he was blind from **birth** - that is he was born blind. The Jews had the belief that for one to be born with a disability, it had to be a punishment for either the sins of his parents or his own sins. That was why the disciples of Jesus asked him "Rabbi (meaning teacher), who sinned, this man or his parents, that he was born blind?" I could imagine that Jesus would have been saying in His mind, If I were to count the sins of everyone against them, the whole world would have been plagued or destroyed by now (If You, Lord, should mark iniquities, O Lord, who could stand? Psalm 130:3). Jesus explained to his disciples that this man's blindness was not as a result of sin - neither him nor his parents; but that the wondrous works of God would be made manifest through the man's situation. And indeed it was! Jesus spat on the ground, made clay with the saliva, anointed the blind man's eyes, and asked him to go and wash in a pool called Siloam. The man obeyed this instruction and received his sight, proving to us that disability from birth can be reversed by God, all to the glory of His name!

Lame and crippled from Birth

Now Peter and John went up together to the temple at the hour of prayer, the ninth hour. And a certain man lame from his mother's womb was carried, whom they laid daily at the gate of the temple which is called Beautiful, to ask alms from those who entered the temple; who, seeing Peter and John about to go into the temple, asked for alms. And fixing his eyes on him, with John, Peter said, "Look at us." So he gave them his attention, expecting to receive something from them. Then Peter said, "Silver and gold I do not have, but what I do have I give you: In the name of Jesus Christ of Nazareth, rise up and walk." And he took him by the right hand and lifted him up, and immediately his feet and ankle bones received strength. So he, leaping up, stood and walked and entered the temple with them - walking, leaping, and praising God.
Acts 3:1-8

And in Lystra a certain man without strength in his feet was sitting, a cripple from his mother's womb, who had never walked. This man heard Paul speaking. Paul, observing him intently and seeing that he had faith to be healed, said with a loud voice, "stand up straight on your feet!" and he leaped and walked.

Acts 14:8-10

We see here two different accounts of two different individuals who were born cripple from birth. Here, it was not Jesus doing the miracles, but his disciples just as He has promised in John 14:12 that if we believe in Him, we will not only do the works that he has done, but that we would do greater works. Peter and John prayed for a certain man that was **born** cripple in the first account. This man was carried and laid at the gate of the temple every day to beg for alms. You know this is what society sometimes thinks is the best vocation for a disabled person, but the devil is a liar; not only is God capable of making them whole, but he is also capable of using them to do great things.

What about you? Have you bothered to look for precedence in the Bible concerning the situation you are confronted with? What is that thing that is happening to you that you think is so strange? My dear, it's not strange and you are not the only person going through that situation. Is it a child you want so desperately? There were more desperate situations in the bible than yours! Are you as desperate as Sarah that she had to let her husband sleep with her maid in order to get a child? Yet as hopeless as their situation was, God finally gave her, her own child! (Genesis 21:2). Your own child will be the next! You just need to believe God's report.

CHAPTER 3

MIRACLES STILL HAPPEN

Jesus said to him, "If you can believe, all things are possible to him who believes."
Mark 9:23

But He said, "The things which are impossible with men are possible with God."
Luke 18:27

A re you in need of a miracle in your life? Well you are not alone in this need, so do I; and I believe everyone needs a miracle in his life in one area or the other. Some people may have need of miracles in an area that is external and obvious to everyone, while some others may have need of miracles in areas that are hidden and known only to them. But no matter the area in which you have need of a miracle, the good news is that miracles still happen and the things that are impossible with men are possible with God. As you make up your mind to begin to believe God for the impossible, you will also begin to experience miracles in your life.

In the preceding chapter, we looked at some miracles that happened in Bible times; some performed by Jesus Christ and others by his followers. I know that many times one can tend to look at Bible accounts as some form of fairy tales that are not capable of happening in our present time. But this is not true, the Bible makes us to understand that 'Jesus Christ is the same yesterday, today and forever (Hebrews 13:8).' This means that the same Jesus Christ that worked miracles in Bible times can still work miracles through us and in us today as we call upon His name in faith.

Triggers of Miracles

I have come to discover that there are certain things that trigger miracles in our lives. The fundamental trigger of miracles is faith. Faith is the absolute belief and confidence in God that He can and will do what He says He would do. The Bible defines faith in Hebrews 11:1 as 'the substance of things hoped for, the evidence of things not seen'. The New Living Translation of the Bible puts it this way: "Faith is the confidence that what we hope for will actually happen; it gives us the assurance about things we cannot see." It is faith that gives me the confidence that the promises that God has spoken concerning my daughter Grace will come to pass. It is this assurance that gives me comfort and also the boldness to challenge you to believe the report of the Lord concerning your situation as well. I am so excited about the miracles that God is about to do that I cannot wait for all of them to happen before I tell about them. That is faith!

If you are already a believer reading this, then know that faith must also be accompanied by a life of holiness for miracles to be triggered in our lives. You cannot live your life in disobedience and disrespect to God and expect Him to use you as His show-piece. This is because God does miracles for His name to be glorified. For the unbelievers God may use certain miracles to draw them to Himself, but for anyone to experience miracles on a consistent basis, then a life of total surrender to God in holiness is inevitable. That is why we often see that when there is a great revival where people are hungry for the word of God and eager to do His will, miracles abound.

As we long to see and experience more of God's miracles in our present time, it would be beneficial for us to also examine notable miracles that have happened in history.

Miracles at Azusa Street
In April of 1906, a great revival broke out at Azusa Street in Los Angeles and this great awakening lasted till 1910. The story of Azusa Street particularly intrigued me because of the numerous

miracles that accompanied this great revival. Most of the miracles that happened at this revival were instantaneous, although there were also few cases that were gradual. Instantaneous miracles are miracles that happen immediately, on the spot; while gradual ones are the ones that happen over a space of time.

There were cases of unbelievable miracles that took place during these meetings, including creative miracles. Creative miracles are supernatural occurrences in which missing or deteriorated body parts are recreated and replaced as new. I was highly inspired as I read of the miracles that happened during the Azusa street revival and I have decided to narrate only some of the creative miracles here as volumes of books have been written on this great revival. I am narrating only the creative miracles here because they are for me, good examples of precedence.

Cut Fingers Grow Out

This miracle happened through Brother Langford. A man who had his fingers chopped off by a machine several weeks earlier had come to the meeting. The man had heard that God was doing miracles at Azusa Street and he came with the expectation to be healed. Brother Langford approached him and boldly told him that God will grow the fingers back and the man gave him the approval to pray for him.

Langford with the support of his wife held the man's hand high in the air and began to pray and the fingers began to grow out. Mrs Langford passed out at the sight of such a miracle and the man stood in shock with his mouth open in amazement. Brother Langford held the man's hand and ran around in joy shouting to everyone present that his fingers have just grown out. Even new nails grew on the fingers and the man was made whole.

Amputated Leg grow out

A man whose leg was amputated and replaced with a wooden leg also came to the meeting and requested that prayers be made for him. He told Brother Seymour who happened to be leader of this revival that the place where the wooden leg is attached to his leg was beginning to get green. Brother Seymour told him that it would be a challenge for God to grow his leg when the wooden leg was still there, the man then removed his wooden leg and stood on his one good leg. Brother Seymour laid his hands on the man and proclaimed "Let thy name be gloried, in the name of Jesus I command this leg to grow out, the green is out, you are healed". That was it, Brother Seymour couldn't preach that night because the miracles spoke for themselves. The audience went wild and the man ran on the platform and around the room, no one could get him to stop rejoicing and praising God. The man's leg actually grew out!

New Arms Appear

A year later, a man who had lost his arm ten years earlier through a work-related accident and the arm had been totally severed at the shoulder came to be prayed for at the revival meeting. Brother Seymour asked the crowd "Would you like to see God have a wonderful time here tonight?" He went ahead to remind them of the miracle of the man's leg that grew out a year earlier. Brother Seymour then asked the man whether he was able to make a living with just one arm and the man replied that he was only given menial jobs and he is barely able to make a living out of it. Brother Seymour on realising that the man was married with kids said "that is not good. This man needs to be able to make a living; he needs to work so as to be able to pay his tithes." He then jokingly asked the man "will you tithe if I pray for you and God heals you?" The man replied "yes". Brother Seymour burst out laughing saying he was just having fun; then he slapped his hands on the man's shoulders and commanded the arms to grow out. The healed man stood in total shock as the arms grew out and he felt it with his other hand. A few weeks later, the man came back with about two hundred people. He testified that he has gotten his full job back and many of the people he brought with him needed healings and they were prayed for.

A new Ear Grows out

Another story was told of a woman who caught her husband in adultery with another woman. She got into a fight with the adulterous woman and the adulterous woman bit off her ear. The woman came to the meeting with a bloody bandage on the wound and was in tremendous pain. A sister by the name, Connie went over to minister to her, she removed the bandage from the wound which looked like a raw piece of bloody meat and began to pray for the woman. After praying for her, the lady said the pain was gone and when Sister Connie looked at the wound again, to her astonishment, a brand new ear began to grow out; even Sister Connie herself was shocked to see what was happening.

Nose Restored as new

There was a case of a woman whose nose has badly deteriorated as a result of cancer. She had to wear a mask over her nose because it looked terrible and did not smell good either. When she came to the meeting, she was prayed for and instantly her nose was restored as new. She got a brand new nose!

The amazing thing is that God used a one-eyed black man by the name of William Seymour to lead this revival! This was at a time when black people had little significance. Our God is humorous! Anyway, this is in line with His word in

1Corinthians 1:27-29 (NLT) '...God chose things the world considers foolish in order to shame those who think they are wise. And he chose things that are powerless to shame those who are powerful. God chose things despised by the world, things counted as nothing at all, and used them to bring to nothing what the world considers important. As a result, no one can ever boast in the presence of God.'

Prophecy by William Seymour

William Seymour gave a prophecy in 1909 that in about a hundred years after the Azusa Street revival, another revival similar, but greater than that of Azusa Street was going to spring up, but this time it was not going to be in one place like Azusa, it was going to be in different places all over the world.

This prophecy is in line with the word of God in Joel 2:23

> *'Be glad then, you children of Zion, And rejoice in the Lord your God; For He has given you the former rain faithfully, And He will cause the rain to come down for you - The former rain, And the latter rain in the first month.*

I strongly believe that the revival recorded in Acts chapter two can be referred to as the former rain, while the Azusa Street revival could be referred to as the latter rain. I am also of the opinion that the former and latter rain coming at the same time as mentioned in Joel 2:23, would be in fulfillment of this prophecy by William Seymour; and thereafter will usher in the second coming of our Lord Jesus Christ. Our responsibility now is to arise and begin to do things that will trigger this revival.

CHAPTER 4

NO MORE TEARS

The tears could not just stop flowing, I was very much devastated. I often wondered whether I would ever smile again. I thought my whole world had crumbled. Looking at my child's condition and the medical report I have been presented with, the future looked very bleak. It was in this state of 'hopelessness' that I was given Lena Maria's book 'Footnotes' by a Christian sister, Yinka Sanni of the Redeemed Christian Church of God, Jesus Centre, Dublin in January, 2004 shortly after I gave birth to Grace. That Book to me was like a message coming directly from God to strengthen me! It did comfort me in no small measure and gave me the courage to believe that God has great plans specifically for my daughter.

Lena Maria was the first person I got to know of that was born with missing limbs after my daughter, Grace. I saw so much similarity between Lena Maria's mum and myself; between her family and mine; between her birth circumstances and that of my daughter. Her parents were committed Christians with a strong faith in God, and so were my husband and I. As a matter of fact, my husband had resigned his secular job and had become a full-time pastor eight months prior to the birth of Grace. She was born around eight o'clock in the morning; my baby was born around eight o'clock in the evening. She weighed only 2.4kg at birth, Grace weighed only 2.08kg at birth. She looked so pale when she was born, and so was Grace. Her mum had to pump breast milk for her to be fed, and this was what I saw myself doing at the time. The first time after her birth that her mum was allowed to go and see her, the mum was pushed in a wheel chair because she was so weak; this was still exactly what happened to me, I was pushed in a wheel chair the day after Grace's birth that I decided to go and see her. The similarities in her birth circumstances and mine were so parallel that it felt like I was reading my own story when I read her book. I knew at that moment that this was more than mere coincidence. God has brought this book my way to confirm His word that "the temptations in **my** life are no different from what others have experienced. And God is faithful. He will not allow the temptation to be more than **I** can stand. When **I** am tempted, He will show **me** a way out so that I can endure. " I Corinthians 10:13 (NLT emphasised and adapted by me and to me).

Lena Maria, thank you so much for putting your story into print; my comforting process started with reading your story. Your story gave me strength and the courage to believe that there is hope for my baby. Your mum's courage in raising you especially inspired me and showed me the way to face the challenge. Your life has taught me that God can either do a miracle in us or make us a miracle for others to behold. Your life and your accomplishments to me are a miracle and a wonder to behold. You have achieved and done things that many of us that are born with two full legs, ten toes, two full hands and ten fingers have not been able to do! It is with this great admiration for you that I want to share some of your success stories here.

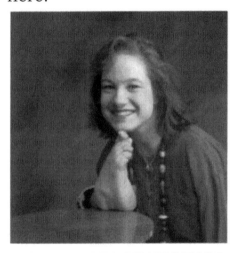

LENA MARIA KLINGVALL

Her Background

Lena Maria hails from Sweden. She was born in Jonkoping Hospital on the 28th September in the early seventies to Rolf and Anna Johansson; both of whom were very committed Christians. News of her birth which should have been a message of joy to relatives and friends became a message of sorrow instead! She is the first child of her parents, after which was born her brother, Olle with no form of disability whatsoever.

Her Birth

Lena Maria was born with no arms at all, where her shoulders finished were just two small stumps. Her right leg is normal, but her left leg is only about half the size of the right one. Because her face was so blue when she was born, coupled with her physical disability, there was very little hope that she would survive.

Her Challenge and Determination

Lena experienced a lot of challenges growing up. A lot of input (especially from her mother) was needed to make her do what most kids would do with ease. Her mum, who was an occupational therapist, had to give up her job the first ten years of her life to raise her; she also had good support from her dad. Her parents' love and support gave her the much needed security she required when she was growing up. She attended a main stream school with the help of an assistant.

For Lena Maria, overcoming her challenges was all about adaptation. She learned to do with her legs what most people would do with their hands. Such things include:

- Counting money with her feet, when sitting down
- Dressing and undressing herself.

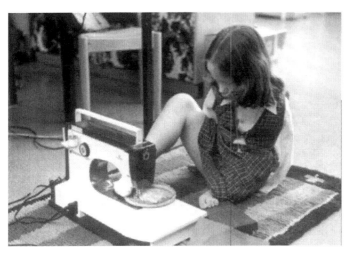

- Sewing

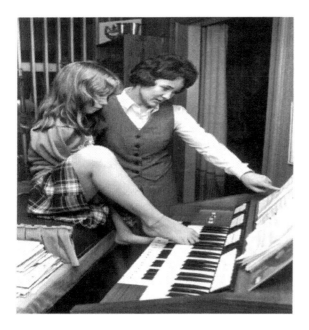

- Learning to play the organ

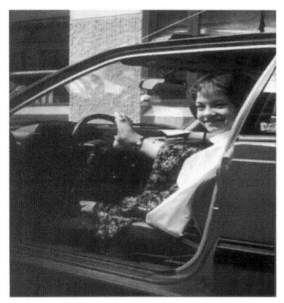

- Driving her own car

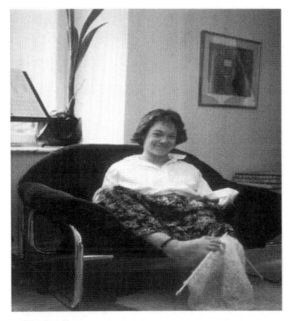

- Knitting

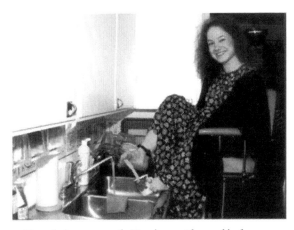

- Cooking and Doing the dishes

- And many other everyday chores that is necessary for living.

Her determination, persistence and faith in God led to some of the achievements mentioned below:

Swimming

She started learning to swim at 3 years of age using the Halliwick method. Her progress in swimming led her to participate in the Swedish Championship for the disabled in 1986 held at Stockholm. In this competition, she participated in 4 different events - 25 metres butterfly stroke, 25 metres back stroke, 25 metres breast stroke and 25 metres free style. She came second in both the back stroke and the free style, in which she won 2 silver medals. In the butterfly stroke, she not only won the competition with a gold medal, but also broke the Swedish record.

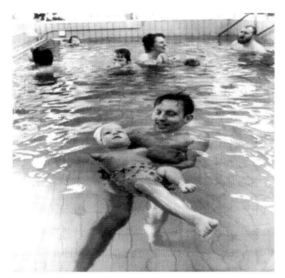

Learning to swim at an early age

This opened the door for her into the Swedish National team for the disabled, which meant she had to take her swimming training very seriously. During her intensive training sessions, she swam between 2,000 and 3,000 metres in every session. She was then chosen to represent Sweden in the World Championship held at Gothenburg in 1986. At this World Championship, she again won another gold medal and a bronze medal.

In 1987, she also participated in the European Championships in France, in which she won four gold medals in four different events. One of such events was the butterfly stroke (her favourite) in which she beat the world record. She later went on to represent Sweden in the Olympic Games for disabled otherwise known as the Paralympic Games in 1988 held in Seoul, South Korea. She was entered for four events - 25 metres back stroke, butterfly stroke, free style and breast stroke. But unfortunately for her, her all-time favourite, the butterfly stroke which she was banking on was cancelled the evening before the event because there were not enough countries that entered for it. She however made fourth place in the back stroke, fifth place in the free style and sixth place in breast stroke.

Music

For Lena Maria, music started at her very early years. As a child, she sang in her local church choir and as she grew, she progressed to the youth choir, where she became the leader. She composed her first song - 'I want to be a friend' when she was a child in the children's choir. While she was involved in music in church, she was also involved in music at school. Even though she was not particularly good at singing, and nobody believed in her voice, she thought music was great and really enjoyed it.

From her music teacher coming to her house once every week to teach her when she was in her third year at school, to her taking music lessons at the community music school in her ninth grade, she continued to make progress with her music. She also progressed to study music at the Per Brahe School's music stream for three years before moving on to Stockholm's Music Conservatory where she studied music for four years. Because of her desire to touch people's lives through music, she worked hard at developing her voice while at the music conservatory with the help of her music teacher. It was while at this college, that her music teacher, Lena Ericsson invited her to sing at GronaLund entertainment Park, where she was also going to sing. At this event, she was chosen by an association for people who are in entertainment, to receive their Bosse Parnevik Scholarship where she was given flowers and a cheque for 10,000 Swedish Kronor to enable her continue her music study. This award was featured in the newspapers, and that made Lena Maria very famous and in no time she granted several TV interviews. Through a documentary that the Swedish television made about Lena Maria, new doors opened among which was the opportunity to meet with the Queen of Sweden - Queen Silvia in 1989, who gave her a scholarship of 10,000 Kronor to continue her study of music. She has released several musical albums.

Author

Lena Maria is also an author. Her first book "Footnotes" which she wrote with her feet was first published in Sweden in 1996. It was later translated to 13 different languages. She published her second book "Happy Days" a few years later. She is currently working on her third book.

Others

Lena Maria attended a 3 month Bible school in Amsterdam, and has had opportunities of engaging in Missionary work in various places including India.

She is also a motivational speaker and has spoken before various audiences including people like Bill Gates. You can get more information on Lena Maria by visiting her website www.lenamaria.com.

Any Hope of Marriage?

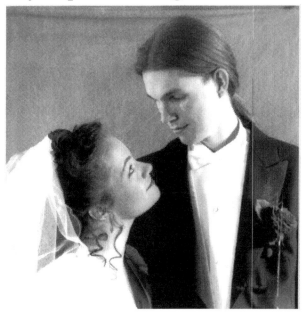

In her book Footnotes, she asked these questions: "can one have a relationship when one is as disabled as I am? If one is to get married, ought one not to marry someone as disabled as oneself in that case? Besides, are there any guys at all that are interested?"* These questions and many others have also crossed my mind when I think of the future of my girl, Grace. However, Lena Maria's life answered that question for me and now, I confidently believe that if we can entrust our lives to God, He knows how to meet our every need, including marriage - yes, even for the disabled!

While at the Music Conservatory, she met Bjorn Klingvall, who was studying to become a music teacher and they became very good friends. They later got married on 1st July, 1995 in the Gustav Vasa Church in Stockholm with over 800 guests present as witnesses. Yes God made it happen! Hear her own words "I had got the husband who was the very best, and the one who had been my very best friend ever. He is the finest person I know and has a wonderful and warm heart. I was happy on that day, and I am still happy, proud and thankful for getting Bjorn of all people."*

In Conclusion

Lena Maria's positive attitude to life is infectious. How can someone who has enough reasons to be negative, critical and bitter towards God and man,

Lena Maria Footnotes Published in Great Britain by Monarch Books 2000

choose to be so positive and achieve so much? She answers this with three reasons:

- Her strong Personality - she is someone who thinks positively and prefers to look at possibilities rather than difficulties. She is a very persistent and determined person. Hear her words when it came to music - "I don't think there was anyone who really believed in my voice to start with, but this did not particularly worry me."

- Her Parents - who created a relaxed atmosphere for her to be comfortable with herself and with people. They did not hide nor fuss about her disability. They loved her and treated her just like any typical child. This she said gave her a very secure foundation.

- Her last and most important reason is her faith in God. She is confident that God loves her and made her just as she is, He couldn't have made a mistake!

The Lord used Lena Maria's story to greatly comfort me and wipe away my tears. I now see that there is hope no matter how hopeless the situation seems. And for people who love Him and put their trust in Him, the end of every situation will be glorious as His purpose is revealed. Through her book, the Lord has delivered my eyes from tears (Psalms 116:8).

CHAPTER 5

I EITHER BELIEVE OR LOSE HEART!

"I would have lost heart, unless I had believed That I would see the goodness of the Lord In the land of the living."
Psalm 27:13

I have come to discover that your life is basically a function of what you believe. Your beliefs determine what you see! If David (the writer of the above Psalm), were looking at his predicament and troubles (which were enormous), he would have lost his mind and even his throne. But he chose to look up to God, the source of his hope and strength which is a sign of his belief in God. No wonder Psalms 121:1&2 says I will lift up my eyes to the hills - From where comes my help? My help comes from the Lord Who made heaven and earth. David knew that the secret of his help from trouble is from the Lord who made heaven and earth. Let's take a brief look at some of the troubles David went through.

The Troubles of David

David was the son of Jesse; he was the youngest of his father's eight sons. He was also a one-time king of Israel who sought and walked with God during his reign as a king and in fact his entire lifetime. He was often referred to as a man after God's heart – 'I have found David the son of Jesse, a man after My own heart, who will do all My will' - Acts13:22. He was not a perfect man; he had several flaws and missed it several times. Yet God was pleased with him, and the Bible makes us understand that he fulfilled his assignment on earth 'David, of course, having completed the work God set out for him,....' - Acts 13:36 (MSG).

David went through so many troubles; yet he chose to believe God in every situation for the best. Talk about someone having challenges from left, right, centre, front and back, and you are talking about David. His challenges, I believe, started right with his own family when he was growing up. He was relegated to just keeping his father's sheep, and being the last son of His father, not much seemed to be expected from him. He didn't seem to be remembered for important events in the family; one of such was when Prophet Samuel visited and asked for all the sons of Jesse to be presented so that one of them could be chosen as king. He was not even remembered! He must have experienced rejection and discrimination in his own family, but despite that, he still joyfully kept his father's sheep in the bush and was eventually chosen and anointed as King of Israel (1 Samuel 16:1-13).

After David was anointed as king, Saul the reigning king at the time developed intense hatred for him. Saul hated him so much that he made several attempts to kill him! All these attempts failed because God was with him. During this period, David never enjoyed peace, he had to keep running from one cave (hide-out) to another; yet he still believed that he would see the goodness of God.

During his reign as king, his lifestyle created a lot of enemies for him. Look at the statement he made in Psalms 69:4 - 'Those who hate me without a cause are more than the hairs of my head.' He had enemies within his household, and enemies externally. Within his household, he had loads of problems with his children to the extent that his son, Absalom conspired against him to take his throne. At this time, he had to run away from his home and his throne, and you can imagine the contempt and reproach he faced as he ran; he was even being cursed and stoned as he fled (2 Samuel 16). But at this time that he was fleeing from Absalom, he still believed God and could still say in Psalm 3:1-4:

Lord, how they have increased who trouble me! Many are they who rise up against me. Many are they who say of me, "There is no help for him in God." But You, O Lord, are a shield for me, My glory and the One who lifts up my head. I cried to the Lord with my voice, And He heard me from His holy hill.

David's disposition towards trouble was amazing! Even when he knew how much his enemies had increased, and the mockery from people who called him a rogue, a blood thirsty man, and said to his hearing that there is no help for him from God; he didn't let that deter his relationship with God. He knew that even though he sinned, he had confessed his sins, and God had forgiven him, so he wasn't going to allow anyone be his judge or a barrier between him and God. He could still say to God - You are my shield, my glory and the One who lifts up my head! And of course you can guess what happened, God actually restored him back to his home and throne and lifted up his head.

Externally, he always had one war or the other to fight with other nations like the philistines, Amalekites, etc. During one of those wars, when David and his men were away from Ziglag (a city where he and his men resided at a time), the Amalekites invaded the city, carried all their wives and children away captive and burnt down the city

(1 Samuel 30). When David and his men returned to the city to meet the devastation that was done, the Bible said they lifted up their voices and wept until they had no more strength to weep. And guess what? All his men turned against him and threatened to stone him if he did not produce their sons, daughters and wives, completely forgetting that even David's kids and wives were also taken captive! No one cared how he felt (especially as a leader) seeing the magnitude of devastation done to his people and his city. Everything seemed to work against him at that time, yet he strengthened (encouraged) himself in the Lord his God.

David went through so much ridicule, rejection, distress and disappointments during his life time. Can you now understand why he said in Psalm 27:13 "I would have lost heart, unless I had believed that I would see the goodness of the Lord in the land of the living." Do you know that the pain of going through rejection and ridicule or disappointments and distress is the same irrespective of the cause of it? I don't know what it is that is causing you pain, or that which is making you to be in despair, but one thing I can confidently tell you is to look up to God. Like David, decide from today that you will continue to look up to God until you see His goodness in your life. And I tell you that very shortly; that goodness will begin to overwhelm you.

Believing means 'Looking Up'

This does not mean you have to walk literally with your eyes looking into the sky. You know you are going to stumble and fall, or have an accident if you do that (Ha ha ha). But I am talking about your inner eyes. Whatever your inner eyes see, in other words, whatever pre-occupies your mind determines the results you are going to receive. If with your inner eyes, you are seeing the seemingly practical impossibility of your situation, as your mind is pre-occupied with the negative things doctors or experts have said; you are going to get very worried, which is a sign of unbelief. But if with your inner eyes you see God fixing your challenges as you meditate on His Word, then hope is going to arise in your heart, making you to believe God. This is what the Psalmist meant when he said in Psalms 121:1&2:

> *I will lift up my eyes to the hills - From whence comes my help? My help comes from the Lord, Who made heaven and earth.*

He had learnt to look up to God, even when surrounded by difficulties and impossibilities. Somebody said you cannot look up and look down at the same time. Can you try it? Try rolling one eye ball to look at the floor, and the other to look to the sky. Was it possible? I'm sure you will agree with me that it was impossible to physically look up and down at the same time. So it is with believing God. Each time you have faith in God through His Word concerning your situation, you are looking up, but when you begin to look at or think about the negative report you have been told concerning your situation, and you begin to worry, you are looking down. Remember this - when you look up, help comes from God, when you look down, distress comes from the devil!

What You Believe and Your Utterances

> *And since we have the same spirit of faith, according to what is written, "I believed and therefore I spoke," we also believe and therefore speak.*
> 2 Corinthians 4:13.

A Christian brother, who had a very major brain surgery, came out of the surgery with some sort of partial paralysis. It was like one half of his body was numb; he could not feel anything even when pricked with a sharp object. But this brother's faith in God for a complete recovery was very strong. As a result of his belief, he refused to utter any negative word concerning his body or situation, and he strongly disagreed with anyone that referred to any part of his body in a negative way. While in the hospital, nurses would often come to him for treatment and say: "Give me your bad leg" (referring to the leg that was numb), even though he understood what they meant, he would often say to them politely - "You mean my left leg?" He refused to agree with them to call any part of his "bad" because he knew the implication of saying that. He knew that whatever he called 'bad' will actually turn out to be bad; therefore he chose his words carefully, even though this did not go well with most of the people around him. This brother was on the wheel chair for a while after the surgery, but he kept saying to everyone around him that he would walk on his feet out of the hospital. Even though this did not look realistic, he actually walked on his feet out of the hospital! Praise the Lord! This is what faith in God can do!

As children of God who believe in His miraculous working power, we need to only say what we believe, and refuse to utter words that contradict what we believe. Sometimes in trying to be "nice" to people, we agree with the negative utterances they make about our situation, forgetting that whatever any two agree on earth, is also agreed in heaven. My daughter, Grace is now eight years old, and does not walk or speak yet. Often when people enquire about her, they would ask: "Does she have any speech?" My reply is usually - "Not Yet", because in my heart I believe she will speak! Or they would ask: "Can she walk?" And my reply is -

"She does not walk unsupported yet", because I know that she will definitely walk.

> *By faith we understand that the worlds were framed by the word of God, so that the things which are seen were not made of things which are visible.*
> Hebrews 11:3

> *By faith - by believing God - we know that the world and the stars - in fact, all things - were made at God's command; and that they were all made from things that can't be seen*
> Hebrews 11:3 (TLB).

The above scripture clearly tells us that visible things are made from the invisible. The words we speak which is invisible is very powerful, and controls the world we live in which is visible. We understand that this is the principle by which God works. In Genesis, the first chapter, we see God demonstrate this principle in creation. There was darkness upon the earth and because God wanted light, He said, "Let there be light"; and light had to show up. Everything God created first happened by word of mouth - His utterances; even the creation of man! Genesis 2:7 says: And God formed man of the dust of the ground, and breathed into his nostrils the breath of life; and man became a living being. But prior to God using dust to form man, He first spoke man into existence in Genesis 1:26 when He said let us make man in Our image. If the God of all, spoke the things He wanted into 'being'- into existence, then we who believe in Him have to do likewise. This is the principle of making things happen for those who believe. If you say you believe the promises of God for your life, then never let your utterance contradict what you believe, but should rather express and confirm what you believe.

*** Remember that there are times that you just speak, and there are also times that your utterances are backed up with corresponding action. FAITH WITHOUT WORKS IS DEAD!

BELIEVING PRECEDES VISITATION

Abraham & Sarah

> *And the Lord visited Sarah as He had said, and the Lord did unto Sarah as he had spoken. For Sarah conceived and bore Abraham a son in his old age, at the set time of which God had spoken to him.*
> Genesis 21:1-2

Everyone who ever had a visitation from God first had to deal with their unbelief. We all experience unbelief at different points in our lives especially when we are confronted with situations that seem humanly impossible. This was the case with Abraham and Sarah before the arrival of their promised child, Isaac. They had their seasons of unbelief which God had to deal with. Due to the seemingly 'impossibility' or impracticability of God's promise to Abraham which was quite difficult to belief and accept (Just imagine yourself still expecting to have a child at 99 years of age, when your wife is 89 years old - difficult to believe you will agree), God had to deal with Abraham's (formerly known as Abram) unbelief in various ways and at different stages.

1. Use of Symbols - In Genesis 15 when Abram got concerned about the issue of his childlessness, presuming that his servant, Eliezar, who was born in his house, was going to be his heir. God stepped in to correct that presumption that the child He had promised Abram was to come from his (Abram's) own body. God kindled Abram's faith by taking him outside and showing him the stars. Genesis 15:5 - Then He brought him outside and said, "Look now toward heaven, and count the stars if you are able to number them." And He said to him, "So shall your descendants be." In Verse 6 (TLB) - And Abram believed God; then God considered him righteous on account of his faith. This is the power of symbols. Abram, who was initially wavering in unbelief, had his faith rekindled by virtue of signs God showed him. Is your faith in God concerning a situation you believe Him for wavering? Then ask Him to show you a sign or give you a symbol that would cause your faith to be rekindled.

2. Change of Name - When Abram waited for some while and the promised child didn't seem to come forth from his wife, Sarai; he agreed with his wife's suggestion to have the child through another woman (Sarai's maid). Abram must have said to himself - "God told me that the child would come from my own body, so having the child through Sarai's maid is still my seed, my own body!" Therefore he went into Hagar and gave birth to Ishmael. Oh how we often tend to twist God's promises when we think time is running out! But God will always be true to His promises. He therefore stepped in again to correct this misconception of Abram and his wife, Sarai. This time around, He decided to change their names, so that as their names are called by various people at different times of the day, it will remind them of His promise. Genesis 17:5 (TLB) - *"What's more," God told him, "I am changing your name. It is no longer 'Abram' ('Exalted Father'), but 'Abraham' ('Father of Nations') - for that is what you will be. I have declared it. Verse 15-16 - Then God added, Regarding Sarai your wife - her name is no longer 'Sarai' but 'Sarah' ('Princess'). I will bless her and give you a son from her! Yes, I will bless her richly, and make her the mother of nations!*

3. Covenant of Circumcision - God told Abraham to circumcise every male in his household. This covenant will also extend to every male child born even later into Abraham's family. The baby is to be circumcised on the 8th day. This was quite a painful experience for Abraham and his entire household. Just imagine going through circumcision at 99 years of age! That must have been an ordeal, an experience that I am very sure, if Abraham had his way, he wouldn't want to go through. But this experience sealed God's promises to Abraham.

After God had dealt with Abraham's unbelief, He also had to deal with that of Sarah, Abraham's wife. In Genesis 18, the Lord appeared to Abraham in the form of three men whom Abraham gladly hosted and entertained. After they had eaten and about to take their leave, the Lord inquired of Sarah, whom Abraham said was in her tent. Genesis 17 (TLB) *10Then the Lord said, "Next year I will give you and Sarah a son!" (Sarah was listening from the tent door behind him.) 11Now Abraham and Sarah were both very old, and Sarah was long since past the time when she could have a baby. 12So Sarah laughed silently. "A woman my age have a baby?" She scoffed to herself. "And with a husband as old as mine?*

Here is Sarah struggling to accept the promise of God and struggling with unbelief. She had waited so long for the materialisation of this promise and it had not happened up till now. Why is God still coming to remind them of the promise again? Especially since she had aged so much and menopause had set in! How can an old woman of 89 years become pregnant with a child for an older man of 99 years? These I suppose were questions she asked, that made her laugh silently to herself. But God who is omnipotent (all Powerful), omniscient (all-knowing) and omnipresent (always-present) saw her in her closet and heard her laugh; even though it was an inward silent laugh of unbelief, yet God saw it! God challenged her unbelief by reminding her that *14Is anything too hard for the LORD?* I guess Sarah must have reasoned within herself that if this God can see me in my tent where I am hiding and hear my silent laugh, and read my thoughts, then I had better give Him a chance at believing again. Therefore she rekindled her faith in God, and both she and her husband believed.

As believing precedes visitation, when Abraham and Sarah believed God, God visited them at the time He had promised.

> *Then God did as he had promised, and Sarah became pregnant and gave Abraham a baby*

son in his old age, at the time God had said; and Abraham named him Isaac (meaning Laughter!") Eight days after he was born, Abraham circumcised him, as God required. (Abraham was 100 years old at that time.)

And Sarah declared, "God has brought me laughter! All who hear about this shall rejoice with me. For who would have dreamed that I would have a baby? Yet I have given Abraham a child in his old age!

Genesis 21:1-8 (TLB)

As you believe God and continue to hold onto His promises, your own visitation will come shortly. Even if all hope seems to be lost, be like Abraham that - even when there was no reason to hope, Abraham kept hoping-believing that he would be the father of many nations - Romans 4:18 (NLT). And indeed he turned out to be!

The Centurion's servant

Then Jesus said to the centurion, "Go your way; and as you have believed, so let it be done for you." And his servant was healed that same hour.

Matthew 8:13

Then Jesus said to the Roman Officer, "Go back home. Because you believed, it has

happened." And the young servant was healed that same hour.
Matthew 8:13 (NLT)

The experience of the Roman officer otherwise called the centurion was another classic example in which God demonstrated that believing precedes visitation. This Roman Officer who had a servant that was paralysed and dreadfully tormented at home approached Jesus to heal this servant. Jesus wanted to come to his house to heal this servant, but the Roman officer who understood authority told Jesus to just speak a word and he knew his servant would be healed. He not only believed that Jesus could heal his servant, but also believed that a word from Jesus was good enough to heal his servant. No wonder Jesus excitingly and openly commended his faith and his servant received a visitation of healing from God immediately.

Even if God does not show you a sign like He did for Abraham, still hold on to His word, because a word from Him can turn your situation or captivity around. Whatever it is, believe, and you will be visited shortly.

CHAPTER 6

IN THE STATE OF WAITING

*If a man dies, shall he live again? All the days of my appointed time will **I wait** (emphasis mine), till my change come.*
Job 14:14 (KJV)

Waiting is something that no one likes to do. When you walk into a shop or go for a doctor's appointment, you don't want to waste your time; (yes we look at waiting time as a waste of time) you want to be attended to immediately. Most especially in this jet age where everything is on the fast side - we have fast food, speed post, express service & delivery, etc. But do you know that waiting time is never a wasted time? Neither should it be an idle time! It should rather be a time of training and preparation; a time of service - call it internship if you like because it is a time when you have the opportunity to gain some practical life experiences. And a lot can be done while you're waiting on God for your miracle to break forth.

One vital asset that we gain during the waiting period is patience. Waiting teaches us to be patient, and patience is a vital tool that is needed to obtain our promise from God. When we have acquired patience, and begin to exercise it, it is a proof that our faith has moved to a higher level.

> *For you have need of steadfast patience and endurance, so that you may perform and fully accomplish the will of God, and thus receive and carry away (and enjoy to the full) what is promised.*
> Hebrews 10:36 (Amp)

From this scripture, we see that patience is a prerequisite for receiving from God, and it is the will of God that we should learn patience. That is why He subjects us to some waiting so as to learn patience. During your waiting period, you will find yourself in one of these states:

Apathy, Anxiety or Anticipation

Apathy

The World English Dictionary defines Apathy as lack of enthusiasm or energy: lack of interest in anything, or the absence of any wish to do anything.

Apathy could be described as 'I don't care anymore' attitude. It is a state where your faith in God has grown so cold as a result of a long wait for an expected miracle or visitation from God. The long wait makes you presume that God is not interested in you or your case. You throw in the towel, that is, you give up, saying to yourself that 'what will be, will be'. You stop believing God and even start doubting testimonies of the goodness of God that you hear people share. It was apathy that made Sarah laugh at herself in Genesis 17:12 when the Lord said she was going to be pregnant at 89 years of age.

Apathy is no surprise to God, because He already said in His word that "Hope deferred makes the heart sick, But when the desire comes, it is a tree of life - Proverbs 13:12." So if God knows that if our hope is deferred, if there is a delay in receiving a promise from Him, our heart could get sick (that is we could give up believing Him and give up in despair), why then does He still allow our hope to be deferred and make us wait?

I strongly believe that a very good reason why God would allow our hope to be deferred and allow us to wait; is to help us learn patience as I earlier mentioned. Another good reason is to build up our strength. "If you fail in the day of adversity, your strength is small - Proverbs 24:10." The natural tendency for man is to go into apathy if his hope is deferred, or there is some long wait. But this should not be the case for the people of faith who do not see with the physical eyes, but with the eyes of the spirit. The people of faith have their spirit connected to the Spirit of God, and even if there is some waiting to do, they receive signals and Grace from the Spirit of God. And they are strengthened even in the days of adversity because they can see light at the other end of the tunnel; therefore their hope is not extinguished. Your tenacity to wait without giving up hope is determined by your spiritual strength. That is to say that the rate at which you give up - throw in the towel in the face of trying moments is a measure of your strength.

Anxiety

The World English Dictionary defines Anxiety as a feeling of worry: nervousness or agitation, often about something that is going to happen. It is something that worries somebody: a subject or concern that causes worry. It is an intense apprehension, or fear of real or imagined danger.

Anxiety is another extreme that most people tend toward when they are confronted with challenges. Anxiety sets fear (**F**alse **E**vidence **A**ppearing **R**eal) in you and makes your challenge look bigger than it really is. It sets your mind at work figuring out how your problem is going to be solved, and when you cannot figure out a solution, you get more worried. Anxiety makes you look only at the natural, making you to forget the supernatural. Even where there are testimonies of what God has done in the time past in similar cases to yours, anxiety makes you think and feel that your case is different. No wonder the Bible says 'Anxiety in the heart of man causes depression, But a good word makes it glad' - Proverbs 12:25. Anxiety can be very deadly. It can paralyse your faith, lead to a nervous breakdown and cause other numerous health problems.

Hebrews 4:3a (NLT) says – 'For only we who believe can enter his rest.' This means that if we don't believe, we cannot enjoy God's rest. And as you know, there is nothing that steals our rest like anxiety. Anxiety will make you have sleepless nights, it makes you lose your joy of the moment, you are not at peace with yourself and it weighs you down. Anxiety is therefore a sign that you are walking in unbelief not faith, because it takes away your rest. Sometimes you see people going from one man of God to another, from one prayer conference to another (these are not wrong on their own), not because of faith, but because they are anxious. Philippians 4:6 tells us to 'Be anxious for nothing'. The New Living Translation puts it this way: 'Don't worry about anything; instead pray about everything.'

Verse 10 of Hebrews chapter 4 went on to say that 'For all who have entered into God's rest have rested from their labours, just as God did after creating the world.' There is great labour in anxiety. You will agree with me that a day full of anxieties is more exhaustive than a day of hard work. This is because anxiety will not only exhaust you physically, but will also exhaust you spiritually, mentally and emotionally.

Verse 11 -'So let us do our best to enter that rest. But if we disobey God, as the people of Israel did, we will fall.' The favour you can do for yourself is to do your best to enter God's rest! Cease from anxieties! It can destroy you faster than you think or realise. To carry on with anxiety and deny yourself of God's rest is disobedience to God. Determine to drop every anxiety at His feet today. His Grace is sufficient for you.

Anticipation

Anticipation means to wait with a hope of change. It is an expectant waiting, where you are looking forward, usually excitedly or eagerly for something to happen. It was anticipation that made Job say in Job 14:14 (KJV) '..... "All the days of my appointed time will I wait until my change come.'

If you are expectant, you would have hope because you know that what you are waiting for is just a matter of time. You would have a good understanding of God's timing, knowing that He makes all things beautiful in its own time - Ecclesiastes 3:11. Being an expectant person means that you would take time to receive a 'word' from God concerning your situation, hold on to that word until it produces the result that you are expecting. You would not give room to apathy neither would you be anxious because you are confident that God is able to do what He has promised. While you are waiting on/for God to manifest in your life or situations, you make preparations. Making preparations for your expected miracle is a sure sign that you are expectant.

We can get a very good picture of being expectant from a pregnant woman, otherwise known as an 'expectant mother.' As soon as a woman becomes pregnant, all she will be looking forward to will be the day she will be delivered of her baby. Therefore all her plans, projections and preparations are centred on this baby. An expectant mother begins to shop for the baby even before the baby is born. She makes preparations for where the baby will sleep, what the baby will eat, what the baby will wear, and so on; even before the baby is born! A pregnant woman does not compare herself with another pregnant woman and say: 'because my tummy is not as big as that of the other woman, or because I am not as big as the other woman, that I am probably not pregnant.' NO! She sees the signs of pregnancy in herself, she feels the movement of the baby within her and she also believes the report of the doctor that she is pregnant. Even before she begins to feel the movement of the baby within herself, she is convinced that she is pregnant!

To be expectant, you need to be convinced! You get convinced as you study the Word report (The Bible) and ask the Holy Spirit to reveal the truth and mysteries of the Word to you. Ask Him to personally speak to you concerning your situation and He will. You can also get convinced as you learn (listening, watching or reading) of God's miraculous acts in the lives of other people. Remember that if he did it for one person, He can also do it for you; 'For there is no partiality with God' (Romans 2:11).

- Are you convinced that 'with God all things are possible?' Matthew 19:26, Mark 10:27
- Are you convinced that nothing is too hard for Him to do? Genesis 18:14; Jeremiah 32:17&27
- Are you convinced that God is personally interested in you and your case? Jeremiah 29:11

- Are you convinced that God loves you and can turn every situation around for your good? Romans 8:28
- Are you convinced that God is for you and not against you? Romans 8:31, 38-39

Once you are convinced about God's capabilities and His promises, then being expectant becomes easy. Be expectant! Don't give up! Wait on God and for God to bring His Word to come to pass in your life. He is a timely God and will definitely show up for you and make your joy to overflow. Again I say wait on God to be convinced and to receive strength not to give up (Isaiah 40:31, Psalms 27:14), and wait for His time (Ecclesiastes 3:11) for your miracle.

CHAPTER 7

WHILE I AM WAITING

How do I make my waiting period to count? If the waiting time ought not to be a wasted time, how then can I make it productive? I once read in Zig Ziglar's book - 'See you at the Top', a story of a man who was sentenced to several years in prison in Atlanta, Georgia for a 'big mistake' he had made. While going to serve the jail term, he told himself that he wasn't going to make a bigger mistake by "serving time" in jail, but was rather going to make time serve him. This sounded ridiculous, but that was exactly what he did! While in jail, he accumulated a small fortune by operating a tailoring shop. He came out of jail a better and wealthier person! This is what happens when you use your waiting time wisely and productively. I can guarantee you that there were people in that same prison who were waiting to be released before they begin to pursue their dreams; but not so with this man. You can make time serve you while you are waiting for your desired miracle or breakthrough from God, so that when it eventually comes, you will have nothing to lose. As for me, I have decided that:

While I'm waiting, I will Serve

"If anyone serves Me, let him follow Me; and where I am, there My servant will be also. If anyone serves Me, him My father will honour."
John 12:26

"Serve wholeheartedly, as if you were serving the Lord, not men, because you know that the Lord will reward everyone for whatever good he does, whether he is slave or free."
Ephesians 6:7-8 (NIV)

Service is the gateway to honour. In service, you recognise that you have a master, and you take the lowly position of a servant. Serving is a humbling thing to do and that is why it touches the heart of God. Whatever capacity you find to serve - be it in church, in the society, or at home; do it wholeheartedly, genuinely and to the best of your ability. Even if you are serving men, serve them as if you were serving the Lord and you will see how God will begin to move into action on your behalf. Service provokes God to action!

I have therefore decided that while I am waiting on/for God, I will continue to serve. I will not relent in my service to the Lord. I will serve the Lord with every physical, mental and spiritual strength I've got. Have you realised that God has so often visited people who are waiting on Him at the place of their service? Look at the case of Zechariah in Luke 1:5-17. Zechariah was a priest that served the Lord faithfully with his wife Elizabeth. It is recorded that they were both righteous, kept all of God's commandments and were blameless before the Lord, yet they had no child and were now very old. Look at verse 8 - 'So it was, that **while he was serving** (emphasis is mine) as priest before God in the order of his division,' verse 11- 'Then the angel of the Lord appeared to him,....' The angel told him that his prayer has been heard by God and that his wife Elizabeth was going to have a baby, who will be named John, who would be great and turn many to the Lord.

Note here that Zechariah wasn't even asking God about his desire for a child when the angel of God visited him. I believe he had prayed before this time, and even though his prayers were still not answered, he still went into the temple and served the Lord, performing his priestly duty. God, who has watched his faithfulness in service despite the fact that time seemed to be running out on him and his wife concerning having children decided to visit him at His appointed time - in the place of service!

There are countless testimonies where the angels of the Lord have come to visit various people at the place where they ought to be serving and the people were not there. A lot of people give up in their service of God because they have not received what they have asked from God. This is the deceit of the devil because he knows you could get your visitation / miracle at the place of service. Mind God's business; and He will definitely not forget your own business.

While I'm waiting, I will Love

> *Jesus said to him, 'You shall love the Lord your God with all your heart, with all your soul, and with all your mind.' This is the first and great commandment. And the second is like it: 'You shall love your neighbour as yourself.'*
> Matthew 22:37-39

It is very easy to confess with our mouths how much we love God and our fellow human beings, but the waiting time is a good time to test and prove that love. Can we still love God and show (prove) that we love Him even while waiting - that is when it seems as if God is deliberately withholding something from you? I believe God uses the waiting time to test our love for Him; to prove whether we genuinely love Him for who He is or for what we can benefit from Him.

John 21:15 - So when they had eaten breakfast, Jesus said to Simon Peter, "Simon, son of Jonah, do you love me more than these?" The Lord needed to be convinced (The Lord knows all things, so He rather wanted Simon and the people around him to be convinced) that Simon's love for Him was not just because He was giving him food and meeting his needs. I believe the Lord is also posing the same question to you and me today - **do you love the Lord more than these?** That is, do you love the Lord more than the miracles of - healings, children, financial breakthrough, Marriage, and so on and so forth, that you want from Him? If you truly do, then that love will show while you are waiting for the manifestation of your miracle.

So while I am waiting, I need to find out various ways I can express my love to God and my fellow human beings. The Lord lays in our hearts various things He wants us to do for Him while we are waiting and often times, these things would be in the area that we need miracles ourselves. What we often do in such circumstances is to shy away from those things and give the excuse that we are not the right candidate for such works. The Lord gave me the instruction to write this book about six years ago. I was very excited when I heard this instruction and actually started writing, but when I turned to look at my circumstances - at my daughter's present condition, I developed cold feet. I thought to myself - how can I tell people to believe God's report while I am yet to see the full manifestation of that report in my own circumstances? I felt that I would be ridiculed and laughed at. This made me push this instruction aside for several years because I felt that I was not the right candidate to write this kind of book; but because the Lord kept impressing the same instruction in my heart each time I pray, that is why I decided to obey His instruction and write this book. One thing I have come to discover with God is that unless His first instruction is carried out, He will not give the second one! For these past years, each time I pray and ask God to show me the way forward, He reminds me of the book that I am supposed to write. He made me understand that as I expose people to the knowledge of His Word, the Comfort, the Help and the Hope that I have received from Him and is still receiving, He would do more for me. If this book is of any help to you, then I believe the purpose for which it is written would have been fulfilled.

For the waiting parent, you may need to prove your love for God and for your fellow humans by loving and caring for other people's children. This may involve teaching children's classes or baby-sitting voluntarily. If you have the resources, you may even provide homes for motherless babies or even go ahead and adopt a child. There is a school of thought that says Christians should not adopt because they say that is lack of faith. I personally believe that what is on your heart when you are adopting, is what matters. If in your heart, you have concluded that because you cannot and will not have a child any longer, then you decide to adopt, then there is lack of faith there. On the other hand, if you believe adopting is a seed of love you are sowing, while you await your own biological children, it then becomes an act of faith and love. There have been numerous testimonies of couples who adopted and shortly after that, had their own children. I know of a particular couple in Abuja, Nigeria who were married for several years without a child. Shortly after they adopted a daughter, the woman became pregnant and had a set of male twins. In less than two years after the male twins arrived, she became pregnant again and had a set of female twins. She then decided that was enough and went for family planning. Despite the family planning, she had another baby boy! Talk about God giving you good measure, pressed down, shaken together and running over when you give to Him (Luke 6:38).

There are a thousand and one ways you can express your love for God and for your fellow man while you are waiting, this will be based on your individual circumstances and convictions. Expression of your love will put a demand on your time and your resources (financial, material, etc.). You can express your love to your neighbours by doing significant things for them (especially things they cannot do for themselves) and meeting them at their points of need. Remember that you may desperately need attention yourself, but as you continue in these acts of love especially in areas that you desperately need love and attention, you are proving the height of your love for God and man. And just remember that God takes note and keeps record. Your act of love will definitely move Him to act on your behalf.

Another way you can prove your love for God and man will be not giving room for envy and jealousy in your life. Refuse to be jealous of people who have what you want to have, but rather choose to celebrate and rejoice with them. As you rejoice with people who are rejoicing, you are sowing a good seed, and in due time, others will also come and rejoice with you. Give no room for strife and bitterness in your life. Remember that love and envy/bitterness cannot go together.

While I'm waiting, I will Train

But solid food is for the mature, who by constant use have trained themselves to distinguish good from evil
Hebrews 5:14 (NIV)

No discipline seems pleasant at the time, but painful. Later on, however, it produces a harvest of righteousness and peace for those who have been trained by it
Hebrews 12:11 (NIV)

The waiting time is a time of Practical experience. It is a painful time when we learn to differentiate good from evil. It is a time when we get to know our true friends. Everyone undergoes some form of pain while waiting - there is the pain of 'incapacitation'; that is not being able to move when you want to, or knowing what to do yet circumstances would not allow you to do it. There is also the pain of ridicule from people around you. However if you realise that the waiting period is a training period, you will begin to learn how you can convert every painful experience into a useful tool that can be used to make you a better person and your society a better place. Talk about turning your lemon into lemonade!

There are also certain skills that you acquire during your waiting time - there is the skill of patience, which is, learning to wait to receive something. There are also so many innate abilities in you that have been dormant, which invariably come alive during your waiting time as demands are placed on them. I never knew that I had the ability to write and I have never received any formal training whatsoever in writing, but my waiting period has activated the writer in me. I began to write as occasions demand and I am gradually seeing this ability turn into a skill. Training is all about learning the necessary skills to do a job, especially through practical experience. Training equips you with the know how to do a job and it does not necessarily have to be acquired within the four walls of an institution.

> *Everyone who competes in the games goes into strict training. They do it to get a crown that will not last; but we do it to get a crown that will last forever.*
> 1Corinthians 9:25(NIV)

Training is also a time of preparation. Before any sports person goes for any competition, he/she takes time to train because training grooms you for the task ahead. Every profession has some training programme in place to groom its students before they are released to go and practice. God therefore uses waiting as a tool to prepare us for the task He has for us. Knowing therefore that the waiting period is a training period, the onus of how productive your waiting becomes lies with you. I have therefore decided that while I am waiting, I will undergo my training productively and consciously.

There is a saying that 'what you believe determines how you behave, and how you behave determines what you become.' Do you believe that a change is coming to your life and circumstances? Then why don't you start training towards handling that change? For the single person who desires to be married, start training to be husband or wife. For the couple who believe they will have their own children, start training to be parents. For the person seeking an employment, keep up with training in relevant courses. Even if you have health challenges, there is still some training that you can embark on while awaiting your complete recovery. As a matter of fact, your training hastens your change process.

While I'm waiting, I will develop my Spiritual Depth

Do you realise that you have a little more time in your life during your waiting period? For instance, I discovered that my so-called 'incapacitation' (in the sense that I was restrained to the house most of the time) during the first few years of the birth of my daughter gave me the opportunity to develop my spiritual strength. I had more time to pray, listen to messages, study the Bible and other books than I have ever had before. Little did I know that the spiritual strength I was developing to sustain me during this trying period, was also a training for my ministry in the future. As I took time to develop my spiritual strength, there were also a lot of revelations about my future that the Lord showed me; and that gave me the stamina to go through any storm. As a matter of fact I developed a spiritual agenda that I followed every day. Apart from the fact that I was growing spiritually, I was also very busy with no idle time at all.

While I'm waiting, I will Rest and Enjoy

Being able to rest in the midst of chaos is a sure sign of faith!

On the other hand, being able to rest in a confinement is also a sure sign of faith. This is because when one is restrained from moving at will, one can become very restless. This is why it is very difficult to rest in prison. Being confined in the prison of life by circumstances beyond one's control tends to make one fidget and restless. But just like every prison sentence has its terms which include the amount of time to be spent there, your present confinement or challenges also has a time limit. Knowing then that you may have to wait for a while before your circumstance is changed, don't you think that the wise thing to do while you are waiting is to rest and enjoy the wait? I can hear you say that this is easier said than done, and I completely agree with you. But on the other hand, the fact that it is easier said than done does not rule out the truth that it can be done. It is a matter of changing your attitude towards the whole situation. It is very possible to rest in prison or in the midst of chaos. Jesus Christ showed us an example in Matthew 8:23-26 when he was in the boat with his disciples and a great storm arose on the sea, so that the boat was covered with waves. But Jesus was asleep (a sign of being at peace and having rest). His disciples on the other hand were panicking and restless. When they woke Jesus from His sleep, He did not join in their panic party, all He needed to do was to address the situation and there was calm.

You may say that was Jesus, how wouldn't He sleep in the midst of storms, after all He is God. So let me also draw your attention to Peter in Acts 12:5-6 "Peter was kept in prison, but constant prayer was offered to God for him by the church. And when Herod was about to bring him out, that night Peter was **sleeping** (emphasis mine), bound with two chains between two soldiers; and the guards before the door were keeping the prison". This was Peter in prison, he was bound, he was in-between two soldiers, there were more guards at the door, he was about to be killed the next day, yet he slept! The rest of mind exhibited by Peter here is amazing. We need to strive to attain this kind of rest, that no matter the storm of life that comes our way, we will still have peace and enjoy rest.

I have therefore resolved that while I am waiting, I will take my rest and enjoy the season that I am in. I will not let any kind of pressure steal my rest neither will I let people pressurise me into doing something that is against the will of God in order to get a fast/quick result.

So while I am waiting, I will keep busy for the Lord. I will not allow any idle moment in my life - because 'an idle mind is the devil's workshop.'

CHAPTER 8

My 'SHAPPE' Is For My Assignment

For you created my inmost being; You knit me together in my mother's womb. I praise you because I am fearfully and wonderfully made; Your works are wonderful, I know that full well.
Psalm 139:13-14(NIV)

D o you know that in the agenda of the Almighty God, no human life is an accident? So many times, as parents, there are times when we have certain children and we say that we did not plan to have them. We refer to the pregnancy that resulted in their birth as an accident. This was the mind-set I had when I got pregnant for our daughter, Grace. We originally wanted three kids, so after the third one, we thought we were over with child-bearing so we were not particularly excited with the news of the pregnancy. But God has used her birth to radically change my mind-set and perspective to the fact that no human life is an accident. This is because I have seen purpose associated with her birth and assignment being revealed as a result of her birth. Now I realise that as a parent, I may say I didn't plan to have a particular child, but God that is the maker of that child planned the birth of that child and specifically has an assignment both for the child and also for the parents of the child.

We see from the scriptures above that every human life was specially knit together by God. He took His time to make every single human being a wonderful and an original master piece. The New Living translation of Psalms 139:14b puts it this way: 'Your workmanship is marvelous - how well I know it.' Indeed God's workmanship which is you and I is marvelous! From now on, begin to appreciate and celebrate who you are and how you look because the one who made you says you are marvelous and wonderful. He knew you (that is the kind of person you will be and what you would look like) before He went into 'production' of you. Nothing about you is a surprise to Him because He made you who you are.

> "I knew you before I formed you in your mother's womb. Before you were born I set you apart and appointed you as my prophet to the nations."
> Jeremiah 1:5 (NLT)

This means that just as any manufacturer has a visual image of a product either on his mind or on paper, before he goes ahead to physically manufacture the product, God also had an image of you on His mind before He went ahead to form you in your mother's womb. He did not only know you before you were born, but He also designated an assignment for your life. In the case of Jeremiah as we can see from the above scripture, his assignment was to be a prophet. God therefore has spelt out an assignment for every one of us here on earth and He has uniquely shaped us to suite that assignment and its job specifications.

Job 10:8 (NIV) says: 'Your hands shaped me and made me.'

I read Rick Warren's book "The Purpose Driven Life" and it was a tremendous blessing to me. In that book he gave an acronym for SHAPE as:

S - Spiritual gifts

H - Heart

A - Abilities

P - Personality

E - Experiences

I not only agree with his explanation of how our 'SHAPE' suits our various purposes, but my own experience has further confirmed to me that indeed, our 'SHAPPE' is for our assignment (extra 'P' added by me). Let us look at each of the alphabets in 'SHAPPE' and see how they suit our assignments.

S-Spiritual Gifts

These are gifts that are given to the children of God (otherwise known as believers in Christ Jesus) to aid them in fulfilling their God-given assignments. These gifts include: word of wisdom, word of knowledge, faith, gifts of healings, working of miracles, prophesy, discerning of spirits, different kinds of tongues and interpretation of tongues (1 Corinthians 12:8-10). The spiritual gift(s) that is operational in your life is usually in line with your spiritual assignment. You would realise that if you are given the assignment of an evangelist (to preach and win people to God), you would usually see the gifts of healings and the working of miracles operational in your ministry because God knows that as the you go out to preach and to win people to Him, you would have need of these gifts as an evidence of the power of God so that people can be convinced and come to Him.

H-Heart

Heart here refers to our inner-most desires. The things that move or interest us; or an area for which we have a soft spot. You will agree with me that some of the things that make your heart beat faster may not move your sister or brother, even if you are twins. This is because your emotional heart beat responds to your assignment and the area of your assignment is the area that moves it to beat faster. Several places in the Bible (Deuteronomy 11:13; 1 Samuel 12:20, Romans 1:9 and many others), we are adjoined to serve the Lord with all our heart. This means that the assignment that God has for us is in areas that move our heart. This is why someone who has an assignment to help needy people will easily be moved by the needs of these people; while some other person whose assignment is to bring enlightenment to people will be greatly concerned about the level of ignorance of people and is moved to do something about it.

A-Abilities

These refer to the natural talents that you are born with. They are the things that you do naturally such as singing, dressing, cooking, talking, writing, etc. Do you realise that some of the things that you do naturally, some people pay to learn how to do it, yet they are not able to do it as good as you would! This confirms the fact that you were intricately and uniquely designed by your creator. Your assignment in life is also in line with what you are able to do, the things that you have the ability for. This is not an excuse to be lazy and shy away from responsibilities because you think you do not have ability in that area. You must also be aware that there are innate abilities in you that you may not yet be aware of. You can never tell what you can do except you try it out especially in a situation that you have minimal or no alternative.

In Matthew 25:14-30; we are told the parable of the talents where three servants were each given five, two and one talent(s) respectively. While the servants that were given five and two talents traded with them and got them doubled; the servant given one talent went and hid his and it produced no increase. This servant who refused to trade with his talent was considered an unprofitable servant and severely punished for hiding his talent or ability. Please put your abilities into use from today as they are given to you because of your assignment.

P-Personality

We have the different personality types such as introverts and extroverts. Introverts are people that tend to have an inward focus and process their emotions, thoughts, and observations internally. They need time to think before responding to a situation, and develop their ideas by reflecting privately. They can be passionate, but not usually aggressive; and they aren't easily swayed by other people's opinions. They tend to be shy and quiet and do prefer to think before they act. Extroverts on the other hand are people whose interests tend to be turned outward. They are usually friendly and outgoing and love being in the midst of people. They are feelers more than thinkers and can easily express their feelings and thoughts.

We also have the different temperaments types such as Sanguine, Choleric, Melancholy and Phlegmatic.

A Sanguine is someone who has a need for a great deal of social interaction and enjoys the company of others. They prefer to be with others rather than being alone, and will actively seek out social contact much of the time. They are jolly, fun-loving set of people. St. Peter was no doubt a Sanguine and an extrovert. At the site of the transfiguration, he was ready to set up three tents to entertain the guests!

A Melancholy is a reflective, deep thinker. Their deep thinking could easily lead them to depression if not channeled positively. A Melancholy tends to be introverted and likes to be alone. Geniuses in most fields will usually fall into this temperament group. Prophet Jeremiah is an example of someone with this temperament in the Bible.

A Choleric tends to be seen as open, friendly, confident, outgoing, optimistic, and tough-minded. They typically will exhibit a good mind for envisioning new projects and is an extrovert of a highly selective nature. They are the group of people usually referred to as 'born leaders'. They are usually task-focused and result-oriented. Apostle

Paul in the Bible is an example of someone with a choleric temperament.

A Phlegmatic is a calm, peace-loving, slow, steady person, who is not highly emotional. They tend to be observers of life rather than doers; and since they take few chances and break few rules, they generally lead safe but boring lives. They tend to be more introverted than extroverted; although may not be as introverted as a melancholy neither as extroverted as a sanguine. John the beloved is an example of a phlegmatic in the Bible.

From examples cited above in the Bible, we can see that God uses all personality and temperament types. Since He made you and wired you to be the kind of person that you are, His assignment for you is also suited to your personality.

P-Physical Appearance

Our physical appearance, that is our physique - our size, height, body frame and how we look entirely has to do with our assignment. By this, I mean that area of your physical appearance that is not controllable by you. So whether you are tall, short, handsome, beautiful or ugly (in the eyes of men, because in the eyes of God every of His work is beautiful) it is because of your peculiar assignment.

We see an example in the life of Esther in the Bible, where God positioned her to be a preserver for the Jews. She attained this position of a queen as a result of her physical appearance (Esther 2:15 (NLT) "...... and she was admired by everyone who saw her.") and God's favour, which caused the king to be attracted to her. However, Esther was very conscious of her assignment and did not let her beauty or position intoxicate her unlike her predecessor Vashti. When a plot to eradicate the Jews was made known to her, she gracefully stood up to the challenge to intervene for them, as she realises that her position in the kingdom could be tied to this assignment "......Who knows if perhaps you were made queen for just such a time as this?" [Esther 4:14(NLT)]. Know therefore that your physical appearance is also linked with your assignment.

The life of Lena Maria considered in chapter 4 and Nick Vujicic which we shall be looking at in more detail in the next chapter have also proved to me that our physical appearance including the body parts that we have or don't have, has to do with our assignment. Lena Maria though born without arms and with just one full leg has impacted millions of people around the world through her music, books and preaching of the gospel of the Lord Jesus Christ. Nick born without arms and legs is also doing great exploits for the Lord. He located the assignment the Lord has for his life and he is graciously filling it. His physical appearance has endeared more audience to him than most preachers in the world. In his own words, he said "I found the purpose of my existence, and also the purpose of my circumstance". He did not allow his physical appearance to limit him but rather discovered purpose and assignment in it.

E-Experiences

Our life is a sum total of the various experiences that we have had. Every experience right from the ones we had as children growing up in various homes or communities, our experiences at schools, our experiences with God and so on all add up to shape our lives. Your perceptions and attitudes about everything in life are usually as a result of your experiences. Every experience, especially in the life of Believers who love God is always in line with divine assignment.

I have however discovered that God uses our most painful experiences to align us with our assignments. This became very obvious to me some years back after we started the church in Dublin, Ireland and the Lord spoke to me one morning from Philippians 1:12 "But I want you to know, brethren, that the things which happened to me have actually turned out for the furtherance of the gospel." When I came and had my baby in Ireland, I did not originally plan to reside permanently but it turned out that because of her condition, the option of residing in Ireland seemed the best for the moment. The situation that I felt was a sought of incapacitation has led to the establishment of the church of God and also to the publicising of the gospel through my writings in local papers, magazines and gospel tracts.

Our Lord Jesus Christ was not spared of painful experiences on His way to fulfilling His assignment. In order for Him to be a merciful and a faithful high priest for mankind, He had to have the experience of sufferings like mankind. Hebrews 2:18 (NLT) - "Since he himself has gone through suffering and testing, he is able to help us when we are tested." Our painful experiences just like that of Jesus Christ, shapes us into useful vessels for the master's use.

God does not waste experience; He uses it as a valuable ingredient in the fulfillment of your assignment. But do you know that you can waste your experience(s)? How, you may ask? Any painful experience that you hide and pretend it never happened is a waste. Any painful experience that you forget along with its lessons is a waste. Any painful experience that others around you have not benefitted from is also a waste! May none of your experiences be wasted from today on in Jesus' name.

CHAPTER 9

This is what God Can Do!!!

As you do not know what is the way of the wind,
Or how the bones grow in the womb of her, who is with child,
So you do not know the works of God who makes everything.
Ecclesiastes 11:5

God is indeed an awesome wonder! His ways and works are usually beyond our human comprehension. No wonder He says that His ways are not our ways neither are His thinking the way we would think (Isaiah 55:8).

- What men think is a misfortune, God turns to miracles
- What men think is a mess, God turns into a message
- What men think is an error, God turns into excellence
- What men think is an obstacle, God turns into a stepping stone

- What men think is a weakness, God turns into strength
- What makes men weary, God turns into wonder
- What makes men to sigh in distress, God makes into a sign

I am about to share the amazing success story of another person who I got to know that was born with missing limbs. This time around, it is a young man by the name Nick Vujicic. I could particularly identify with Nick because apart from the fact that he shared something in common with my daughter, Grace (missing limbs), his dad also shared something in common with my husband being a pastor. I find Nick's life exceptionally inspiring because despite not being born with any arms or legs he has accomplished and is still accomplishing great things.

NICK VUJICIC

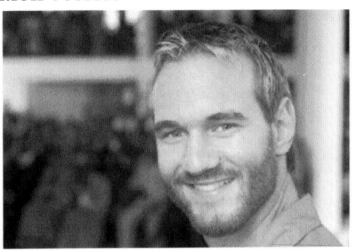

His Background

Nick Vujicic was born in Brisbane, Australia on the 4th December, 1982. He is the first born son of his parents (Nurse Dushka Vujicic, and her husband Pastor Boris Vujicic) who were very committed and dedicated Christians, his father being a pastor of their local Church. His birth was a great devastation to his parents and the entire church; instead of joy it was rather mourning at his birth! 'How could something like this happen to not just anyone, but to a pastor, a servant of God?' Many wondered.

Nick's parents had two other children (a boy and a girl) after him, who were born with complete limbs like any typical child.

His Birth

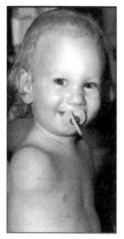

Nick was born without limbs - no arms and no legs at all! Doctors could not give any medical explanation for his birth 'defect' and tests carried out on him showed that he was a healthy little boy with just a few missing limbs.

His Challenge

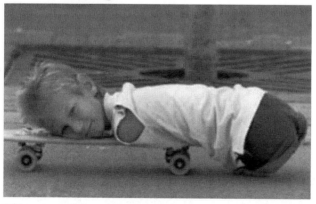

When Nick was of school age, the law in Australia did not permit physically disabled children to get into main stream schools. His mum had to fight this law to be changed and Nick eventually went to a mainstream school.

Nick experienced some forms of rejection and bullying by other students which affected his self-esteem and made him very lonely at school. He constantly questioned why he was different from all the other kids surrounding him; why he was the one born without arms and legs. He wondered what the purpose behind his life was, or if he even had a purpose. His parents however, gave him a lot of support that helped him to develop a positive attitude. They told him that though he was different physically, on the inside he was just like anyone else.

So many times Nick felt depressed and angry with himself. He felt he was a burden on everyone, and felt that the sooner he died, the better it would be for everyone. He found it difficult to reconcile God's message of love to himself, because he would often wonder; "if God loved me, why did He make me the way I am?" But his parents and family encouraged him.

His Determination
Thank God Nick encountered the Lord Jesus Christ at the age of 15 and completely yielded his life to the Lord. After this encounter, he totally believed that God will heal him so that God's name would be

glorified and His awesome power made known. But he later understood that God has a purpose for him and that God's glory can still be revealed by God using him the way he is. He then determined that he would use his experience to help others cope with whatever challenge they had in life by sharing his story. His determination not to hide his pain, but rather to share the love of Christ even in his circumstances has paid off in no small measures. Millions of people have been drawn to the Lord through Nick's testimonies.

Education
Nick is a graduate of Griffith University in Logan, Australia where he obtained a double Bachelor's degree in Accounting and Financial Planning.

His Accomplishments

Motivational Speaker
Nick is a motivational speaker and has a passion to reach out to young people.

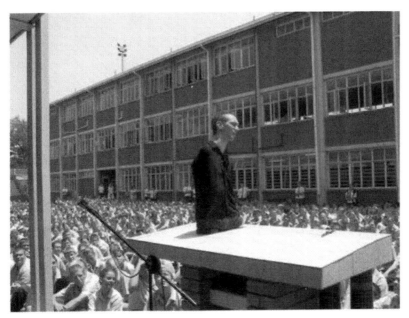

Picture of Nick addressing young students

He also speaks to corporate organisations.

Author

Nick's first book is titled "Life without Limits". In this book, he tells the secret of his passion for life. Nick also released his second book titled 'Unstoppable' in October, 2012. In this book, he tells how being unstoppable is about believing and achieving. It is about believing in yourself, your talents and your purpose and most of all, in God's great love and His divine plan for your life. You can order his books from his website: www.lifewithoutlimbs.org

Mission

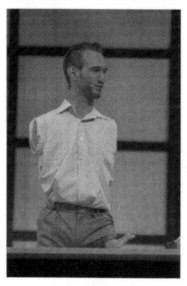

Nick has a passion to share the hope and genuine love of Jesus Christ that he has personally experienced with people all over the globe. At less than 30 years of age, he has travelled to over 43 countries where he has been presented with the opportunity to share his testimony with millions of people and introduce them to the Lord Jesus Christ.

His Marriage
Nick got married to a lovely lady, Kanae Miyaharaa on the 12th February, 2012. Their wedding was celebrated by the world as the wedding of the century.

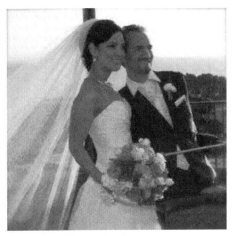

Nick & His wife, Kanae

Others

Nick runs a monthly magazine titled "No limbs No limits". His life is a great inspiration and a source of encouragement to many. He has been able to accomplish at less than 30 years of age, what many people are not able to accomplish in a life time.

Conclusion

A word from Nick: "If you have the desire and passion to do something, and if it is God's will, you will achieve it in good time. As humans, we continually put limits on ourselves for no reason at all! What's worse is putting limits on God who can do all things. We put God in a "box". The awesome thing about the Power of God is that if we want to do something for God, instead of focusing on our capability, we should concentrate on our availability for we know that it is God that works through us and we can't do anything without Him. Once we make ourselves available for God's work, guess whose capabilities we rely on? God's!"

A word is enough for the wise. Stop placing limits on yourself and especially on God. I believe Nick's story has challenged you to live above limits.

CHAPTER 10

NOW I CAN TRULY SAY THANK YOU

"For I know the plans I have for you, declares the Lord, plans to prosper you and not to harm you, plans to give you hope and a future."
Jeremiah 29:11(NIV)

God has really given me comfort. When I look back now, I can truly say "Daddy thank you" for allowing me to go through all that I went through. My experience has helped to shape me better for His service and it has also helped to adjust my values. Some of the things that used to matter so much to me do not really matter anymore. For instance, what people thought or said about me would have been a great deal to me nine years before now and I would not have or have done so many things based on what people would say. But to be honest with you, people can say or think whatever they want to, but what God thinks and says about me is what my heart now yearns for and that is what I am all set to do.

Do you know that in the first year of Grace's birth, I could hardly afford to expose her hands openly because of strange looks and comments from people? Thank God for the cold weather here and thankfully, she was even born in the winter so I would wrap her all up when I am going out not just because of the cold, but also because of people. But as winter gave way to summer, there was no more any hiding place for me; I had to wear light clothes for her which means that she would be seen as she is. A typical Irish person will see her with me and will stylishly come over for a conversation by first remarking - "Isn't she gorgeous? Now tell me, how old is she?" When she was six months and I say so, they would say, you mean six weeks? When I emphasise six months, they would quickly say "Oh she is beautiful" and go their way. But most people of my colour would see us and stare at us strangely, and sometimes when their child tries to play with Grace, they would quickly move the child away.

This attitude from people made me dread going out with her initially. I would pray each time I am going out that no one would ask me about her age or any other such questions, but as soon as I step out, the questions would start coming. So many times, comments from people would make me weep when I am in my closet. But do you know what? Now that I have become strong and those comments don't matter any longer, the comments automatically stopped on their own accord! Now I am the one that likes to initiate a conversation about her. People no longer seem to notice that she has some difference from them. God used the whole process to toughen me and when that was accomplished, He shut the eyes of people from seeing her difference. Daddy, for the strength you have built in me as a result of all these, I say thank you.

For Hope and Faith

My faith has also blossomed over these years. I have fallen more in love with the Lord because He has given me hope. He has shown me light at the other end of the tunnel and I know that in as much as He would perfect all that concerns Grace, He has also set me up to bless me. One of the things the Lord told me shortly after her birth was that He allowed this to happen "that He might humble me and test me, to do me good in the end"(Deuteronomy 8:16b). I believe I have been humbled; I also believe that I have passed my test as I did not give room for bitterness or resentment towards God or any man. I know that now is the season for my blessing, for the good that He promised me. I therefore say that I am truly thankful that God trusted me enough to give me this test. Of course He knows the end of all things right from its beginning, and it is because He knows that I will not disappoint Him that He gave me the test.

I am also thankful because I know that He has great plans for Grace. He has assured me that He has plans to prosper her and give her hope and a future. I am truly thankful to God because I know that her future is bright.

For my family

I am also truly thankful for the kind of husband and children that God has given to me. The birth of Grace has united the family even the more and she is so loved by everyone in the family. She is everyone's pet and thank God for her size, even her immediate elder sister can carry her and take care of her. Sometimes her siblings even fight for who would carry her; and you need to see them defend her when someone makes an unfriendly comment about her.

The children initially asked a lot of questions about why their sister was different, but as we told them that God created her like that so He can manifest His glory through her, they have now come to fully and happily accept her. In fact, one of them recently remarked, "If God gave Grace new arms, I would wonder if she is the same sister that I know". The whole family is now eagerly waiting to see the manifestation of God's glory in her life. I remember that this was one of the things The Lord said to me when she was born. He said that 'This has happened so that His name would be glorified'. I absolutely believe that God would glorify His name in Grace's life!

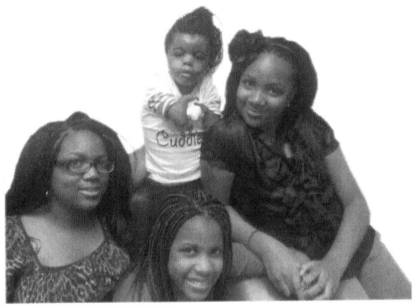

Grace and her sisters

For the People of Ireland

I am also truly thankful to God for the people of this great nation, Ireland. I am grateful that God brought me here to have this baby. Right from when she was born until now, the people of Ireland have been very supportive. They have given me so many privileges all because of Grace. They have ensured that she gets the best of all that she needs, many times at their own expense. I sometimes imagine what my life would have been like had I had Grace in my home country. The all-knowing God that knows the end from the beginning ordered my steps to Ireland and for that I am truly thankful.

For the work of the Ministry

The birth of Grace that kept me in Ireland and subsequently led to the rest of my family joining me here has helped in the spread of the gospel of the Lord Jesus Christ. When I look at souls that have been saved as a result of our ministry, I can truly say I thank you Daddy that you allowed all this to happen. Like Apostle Paul in the Bible, I can also say that I want you to know, brethren that the things which happened to me have actually turned out for the furtherance of the gospel (Philippians 1:12). And that to me is an awesome privilege.

CONCLUSION

Surely there is an end and thy expectation
shall not be cut off
Proverbs 23:18(KJV)

I have shared my story with you so that you may also be comforted. Receiving comfort from God is a sign of assurance of faith. It is a proof that you believe God and that He is in absolute control of the affairs of your life. The bible says of Hannah, after she had poured out her heart to the Lord in requesting for a child that she went back and began to eat again and she was no longer sad (1 Samuel 1:18). She was comforted after she earnestly prayed to the Lord because she believed that God had heard her prayer. Before now, her husband's other wife, Peninnah would taunt her, reducing her to tears that she would even refuse to eat (1 Samuel 1:7). But after she received comfort from the Lord, the taunting did not matter anymore and shortly after, she received her miracle from the Lord, she became pregnant!

I encourage you to earnestly pray to God about your situation and after that, be comforted. God is a faithful God and He will do what He has promised to do in His word. Whatever you are believing him for will surely come to pass and just like He has rightly said in His word, your expectation shall not be cut off.

The New International Version puts it beautifully this way:

> *"There is surely a future hope for you, and your hope will not be cut off"*
> Proverbs 23:18.

Are you saved?

Dear Friend, are you aware that in as much as miracles are good, that the salvation of your soul is better? Whatever miracle you receive right now, can only last for the duration of your life here on earth which at most cannot be more than 120 years. Do you not agree with me that the salvation of your soul is the greatest miracle that you can receive? This miracle secures your eternity where you will live for forever. Why don't you secure that eternity with God? If you want to do so please say this simple prayer:

"Lord Jesus, I believe that you are the son of God and died to pay the penalty for my sins. I acknowledge that I am a sinner and cannot save myself. I confess all my sins (you can mention all

known sins) to you and ask for your forgiveness. Please come into my heart and be my saviour and Lord. Thank You for saving me, Amen."

If you have sincerely said this prayer, then you are now saved and have become a child of God. This is because the word of God says in Romans 10:9 that if you confess with your mouth the Lord Jesus and believe in your heart that God has raised Him from the dead, you will be saved.

If you said this prayer or this book has blessed you in any way, please feel free to contact me at the address below:

Impact Life Publisher

62A Airlie Heights,

Lucan, CO. Dublin

Republic of Ireland

Tel: +353-876408570, +353894895550

Email: info@hegavemecomfort.com

You can also order more copies of this book at: www.hegavemecomfort.com or www.amazon.com

Many thanks and God bless you.

Appendices

APPENDIX 1

Professor Green's Letter

**NATIONAL
CENTRE FOR
MEDICAL
GENETICS**

Our Lady's Hospital for Sick Children
Crumlin, Dublin 12, Ireland
Tel + 01 4096298 / 4096739
Fax + 01 456 0953

DIRECTOR
PROF. ANDREW GREEN, MB, PhD, FRCPI, FFPATH(RCPI)

Ref: 0744/CH
TSCH Ref: 355917/CH

14th Sept 2004

Mrs. Ocheola-Oki
Glenview House
Glenview Lawns
Balrothery
Dublin 24.

Dear Mrs. Ocheola-Oki,

It was a pleasure to meet you with your daughter Grace in the Genetics Clinic. As you know Grace has Cornelia De Lange syndrome, and I enclose a leaflet on the condition which I hope you will find of help.

From a genetic point of view this is a new genetic event which has arisen in Grace and is not something either you or her father would carry. Had you been considering further children the likelihood of a another child with similar problems to Grace would be very small. In relation to your three elder daughters the likelihood of them having a child with Grace's problems would also be very small. If having children for Grace herself becomes an issue then there would be a 50:50 chance for her children of having some form of De Lange syndrome.

I have written to Prof. Matthews in the Rotunda to let him know of our meeting. I haven't specifically arranged to see you again but would be happy to do so in the future should you so wish.

Yours sincerely

PROF. ANDREW GREEN, MB., PhD, FRCPI, FFPath (RCPI)
PROFESSOR OF MEDICAL GENETICS

APPENDIX 2:

Referencing of Bible Quotations

All Bible quotations, except otherwise mentioned are taken from the New King James Version.

Quotations noted AMP are taken from the Amplified® Bible

Quotations noted KJV are taken from The Authorised King James Version

Quotations noted MSG are taken from The Message

Quotations noted NIV are taken from The New International Version

Quotations noted NLT are taken from the New Living Translation

Quotations noted TLB are taken from The Living Bible

Made in the USA
Charleston, SC
24 March 2013